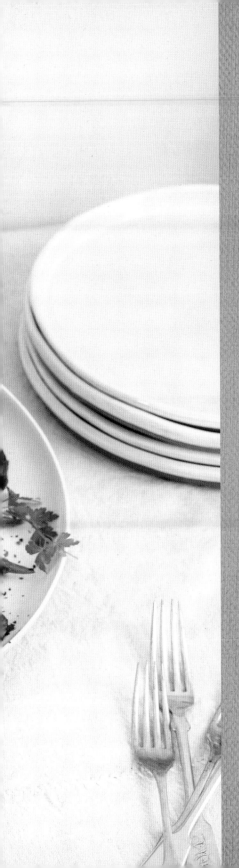

Bountiful Cooking

Wholesome Everyday Meals to Nourish You and Your Family

AGATHA ACHINDU

Food photographs by Rinne Allen

Front cover photograph by Andrew Thomas Lee

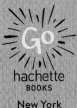

Go

hachette
BOOKS

New York

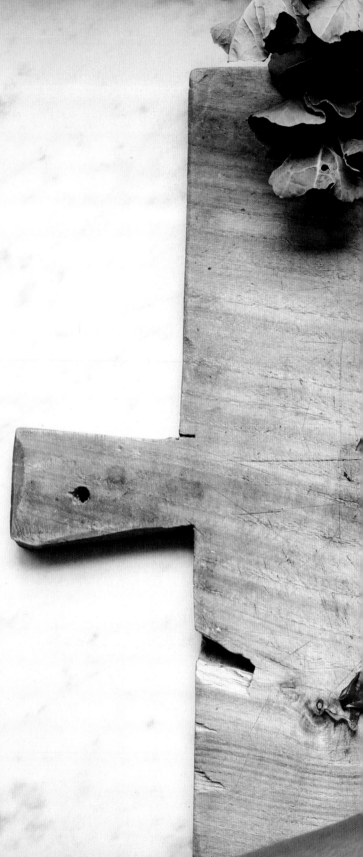

Copyright © 2023 by Agatha Achindu
Interior photos © Rinne Allen

Cover design by Terri Sirma
Cover photograph by Andrew Thomas Lee
Cover copyright © 2023 by Hachette Book Group, Inc.
Print book interior design by Shubhani Sarkar, sarkardesignstudio.com

Hachette Go, an imprint of Hachette Books
Hachette Book Group
1290 Avenue of the Americas
New York, NY 10104
HachetteGo.com
Facebook.com/HachetteGo
Instagram.com/HachetteGo

First Edition: September 2023

Hachette Books is a division of Hachette Book Group, Inc.
The Hachette Go and Hachette Books name and logos are trademarks
of Hachette Book Group, Inc.

The Hachette Speakers Bureau provides a wide range of authors for
speaking events. To find out more, go to hachettespeakersbureau
.com or email HachetteSpeakers@hbgusa.com.

Hachette Go books may be purchased in bulk for business, educational,
or promotional use. For information, please contact your local bookseller
or Hachette Book Group Special Markets Department at:
special.markets@hbgusa.com.

The publisher is not responsible for websites (or their content) that are
not owned by the publisher.

Library of Congress Cataloging-in-Publication Data
Names: Achindu, Agatha, author.
Title: Bountiful cooking : wholesome everyday meals to nourish you and
your family / Agatha Achindu.
Description: First edition. | New York : Hachette Go, [2023] | Includes
    index. | Summary: "Integrative nutritionist and beloved home chef Agatha
    Achindu shares 100 nutrient-dense recipes, inspired by her childhood in
    Cameroon, to nourish the whole family and promote long-term wellness"
    —Provided by publisher.
Identifiers: LCCN 2022045637 (print) | LCCN 2022045638 (ebook) |
ISBN 9780306827204 (hardcover) | ISBN 9780306827211 (ebook)
Subjects: LCSH: Cooking. | Cooking (Natural foods) | Nutrition. |
LCGFT:
    Cookbooks. Classification: LCC TX714 .A3765 2023 (print) | LCC
TX714 (ebook) | DDC   641.5—dc23/eng/20220926
LC record available at https://lccn.loc.gov/2022045637
LC ebook record available at https://lccn.loc.gov/2022045638

ISBNs: 978-0-306-82720-4 (paper over board);
978-0-306-82721-1 (ebook)

Printed in China

IM

10 9 8 7 6 5 4 3 2 1

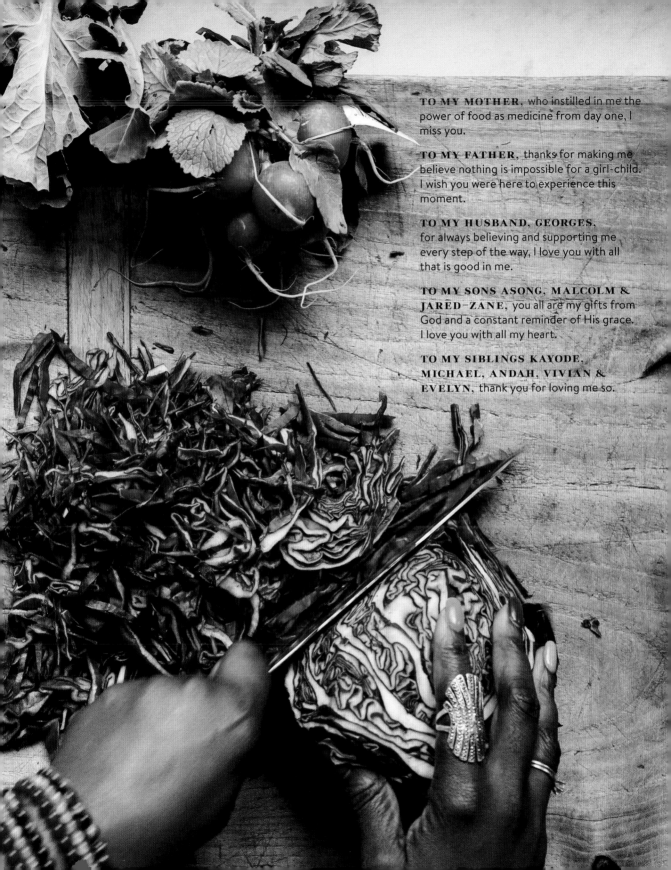

TO MY MOTHER, who instilled in me the power of food as medicine from day one, I miss you.

TO MY FATHER, thanks for making me believe nothing is impossible for a girl-child. I wish you were here to experience this moment.

TO MY HUSBAND, GEORGES, for always believing and supporting me every step of the way, I love you with all that is good in me.

TO MY SONS ASONG, MALCOLM & JARED-ZANE, you all are my gifts from God and a constant reminder of His grace. I love you with all my heart.

TO MY SIBLINGS KAYODE, MICHAEL, ANDAH, VIVIAN & EVELYN, thank you for loving me so.

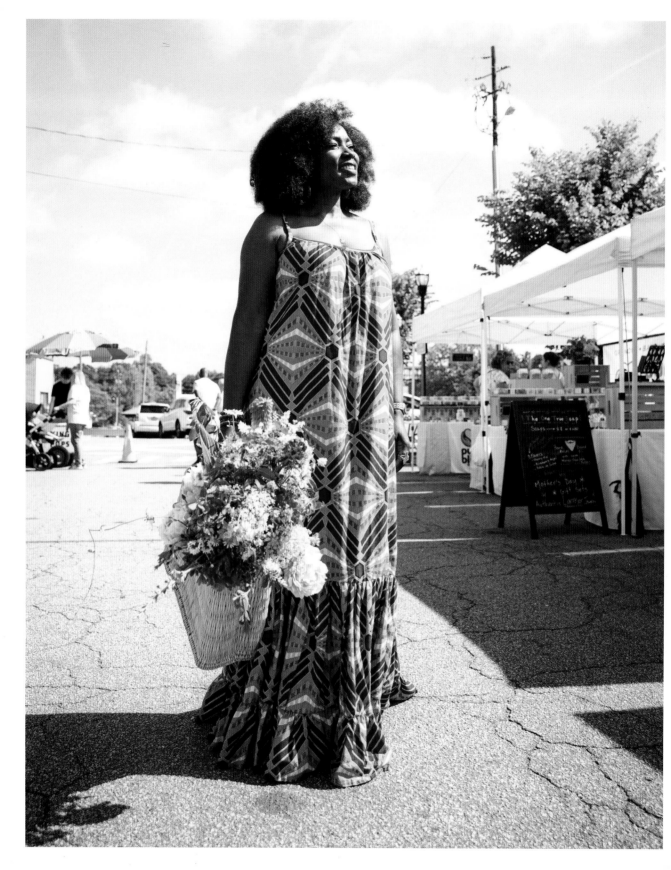

CONTENTS

THE RECIPES

Breakfast

Portable Lunches

Snacks and Treats

Mains | MEAT

Mains | SEAFOOD

Mains | VEGETARIAN

Sides

Nut Milks and Other Beverages

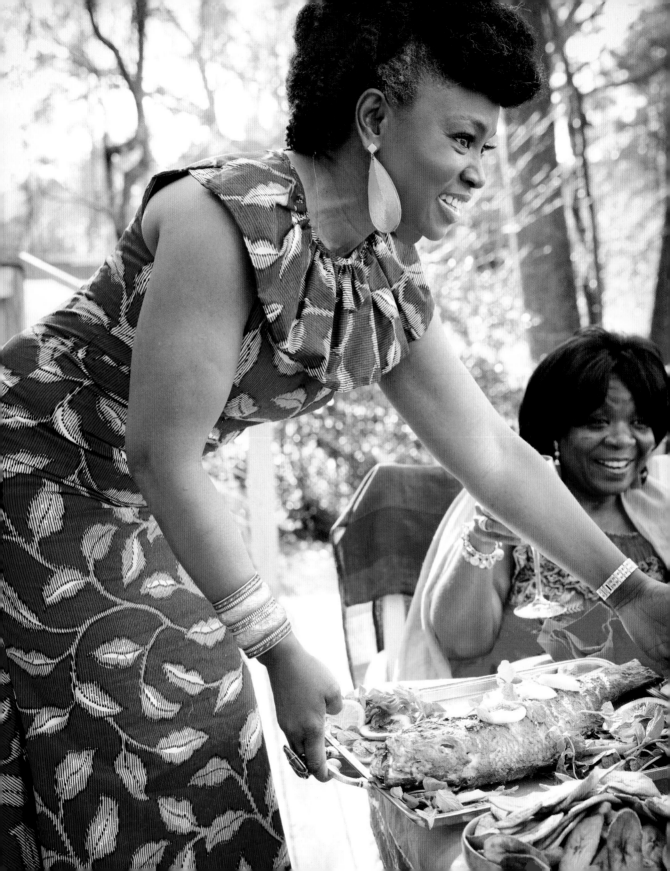

INTRODUCTION

My Story

MY MOTHER'S FARM IN CAMEROON, IN WEST Africa, where I grew up, was a wonderland of natural delights. From the time we could walk, my siblings and I followed our mother around as she pulled weeds and picked corn, beans, tomatoes, and pumpkin. My earliest taste memories involve stolen bites of fresh vegetables, warmed and ripened by the sun. Those early experiences set my eating habits for life.

One of my mother's favorite phrases was "You are what you eat." I am sure you have heard that before, but have you ever truly thought about what it means? For me, the statement is a crucial part of who I am as a woman, wife, mother, and cook; it is also the ethos behind my health- and nutrition-based business. Repeated throughout my childhood, those words instilled in me the fundamental belief that the fuel we put in our bodies is inextricably connected to our overall wellness. My mother truly lived a health-focused life, and I can still hear her voice like it was yesterday:

> "You can't have that Top (a brand of soda)— too much sugar is bad for you."
>
> "Don't throw that plastic in the garden; it will affect the crops."
>
> "Go drink more water; that might be the reason for your headache."
>
> "We cannot use chemicals in the garden because that bad chemical will get in our food."

Our meals were made from scratch every day using ingredients either from our backyard garden, our larger farm, or the twice-weekly, local farmers market. Although we ate mostly plants, my father would get fresh fish from Victoria about once a month. My mother would smoke some of it and freeze the rest. Beef was bought from the butcher on Saturdays to be used for Sunday dinner, holidays, or birthdays. We reared our own chickens, goats, and pigs, which we slaughtered when needed. The refrigerator was mainly for drinks, butter, seasonal fruits, and the occasional jam.

For breakfast, Mami would typically make fried sweet plantains (Sweet Plantains and Eggs, page 62), scrambled eggs with tomato and onions, puff-puff (a super-simple dough made of flour, yeast, a little sugar, and salt and fried to perfection), and pap (fermented corn) or serve fresh bread from the local baker with boiled or scrambled eggs, butter, sardines, or avocado. Lunch would be plantains and a simple stewed vegetable or koki beans (a mashed black-eyed-pea mixture with a fluffy, bread-like texture steamed in plantain leaves with spinach, onion, pepper, and palm oil). Dinner was often fufu, a traditional dish you find across the continent of Africa in various versions and names. It has a dough-like consistency and is usually made from starchy vegetables or grains, such as cassava, plantain, yams, corn, or rice, that is boiled, pounded, and shaped into warm balls and served with soup. The soup (what we call soup in the Western part of the world is typically served as an appetizer or with a main dish, whereas our soups are the main dish served with a side) can be made with just vegetables or with meat added. Fufu with soup is usually eaten with our fingers: you cut a small piece of the fufu, and using a few fingers press it deep in the soup bowl, and then eat it.

When fruits were in season, we would eat as much as our bellies could handle. Mangoes, soursops, guavas, and sugarcane (which is not a fruit but *is* super sweet) were my favorites; we would wait underneath the trees for the mangoes to fall, something that happens when they are just perfectly ripe. Sometimes we were impatient, and we would climb up the tree and gently shake it. (This was totally against the rules.) A cascade of tree-ripened mangoes would fall everywhere— oh, the joyful squeals, under our breath, as we tiptoed, picking as many as we could carry in our dresses, and found a quiet corner and ate until we got tired! That was how simple snacking was. During corn, plums, and peanut season, snacks took a little more cooking effort. There were occasional treats, such as chin chin (fried dough), coconut sweet (thinly sliced roasted coconut and sugar), or chocolate, mainly on holidays and special occasions like birthdays and church feast days. Cake was for Christmas and birthdays only.

Food was simple; it was community; it was love; it was family; it was happiness. Food was the thread that brought everyone in the community together; it was where you found laughter regardless of what was going on. On weekend evenings or during other celebratory occasions, families and neighbors would cook and eat together. I can still hear the laughter and sometimes the tears around the table or the floor where we would gather to eat. Food wasn't broken down to nutrients. We ate what was in season. Every part of a slaughtered animal was eaten, the meat, the skin, the organs, and entrails. My favorite treat as a kid was the juicy, fatty marrow Mami would shake out of the cooked bones for us to enjoy while she used the broth to make jollof rice. I lived for that succulent, warm, jelly-like marrow. And there was no such thing as professional nutritionists and dietitians advising us on what to eat, although basic nutritional information was passed down from the elders when needed.

In 1990, when I was twenty-three years old, I moved to Silver Springs, Maryland, to continue my education. Oh, the excitement when I got my visa! I couldn't wait to come to the United States. As much as I loved growing up in Africa, I thought everything would be better in America. Based on pictures I'd seen in magazines, I believed the houses were large, the roads were paved, the lawns were plush, the models were beautiful, and the grocery stores were filled with all kinds of food. I remember telling my best friend, Clara, how I would make sautéed shrimp with fresh tomatoes, onions, and parsley when I got to the U.S. since shrimp were expensive at home and hard to get.

Well, when it came to the food, the reality was quite different from what I had imagined. I remember walking into a grocery store with a housemate and being greeted by rows and rows of packaged items. I had never seen such massive quantities of canned, jarred, and

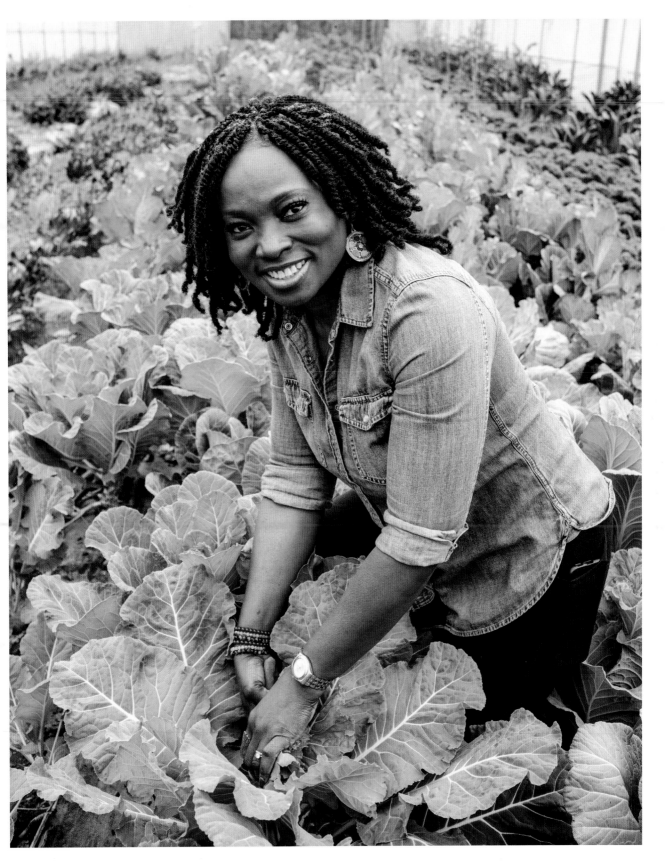

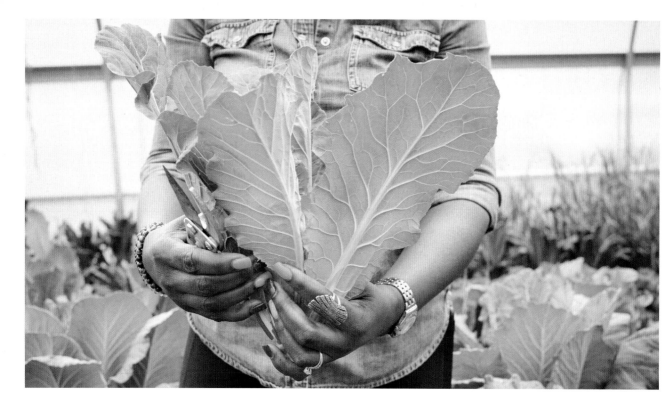

frozen items: beans, corn, peas, fruit cocktail, Mandarin orange segments, mac and cheese, soups, pizza, TV dinners. I asked my friend where the fresh produce was, and she took me to a little corner that housed a few baskets of apples, pears, potatoes, onions, broccoli, tomatoes, and pineapple. That was it.

I was confused. Why would anyone buy corn from a can with a two-year shelf life when you could have fresh corn on the cob? (To be fair, it didn't take me long to understand the value of convenience foods.) I wasn't used to packaged foods, and many of them were outside of my budget, so I made my own food.

Much to my surprise, word began to spread about my delicious, healthy recipes—and my skin. It seemed I was the only twenty-three-year-old without acne or other skin issues. When a friend said she didn't understand why

her skin wasn't glowy, I gently asked her if it could be the fried foods she constantly ate. Then I showed her how to bake juicy, crispy chicken that rivaled the deep-fried version she loved, and she was hooked. Soon, friends and friends of friends were coming to me for simple, wholesome recipes, informal cooking classes, and dietary advice. Newcomers didn't need my address; people joked, "Just follow the sweet smell of sautéed onions to Agatha's apartment." For more than fifteen years I worked with families to implement sustainable eating plans that nourished and brought joy into their homes. In 2006 I founded Yummy Spoonfuls, the very first nationally distributed frozen organic food for kids, to make healthy, affordable, and convenient options accessible to busy parents like me. While I understood that nutrition is the cornerstone of good health,

I was beginning to realize there was more to health and well-being than what we eat, that things like exercise, stress, relationships, spiritual life, environmental toxins, sleep, and genetics all have an impact on our minds and bodies. And that was really the start of my journey toward becoming an integrative nutrition health coach, helping people alleviate or solve common health problems via lifestyle choices and the food they eat.

I went on to study at the Institute for Integrative Nutrition, receiving my health coach certification in 2016. I continued working with individual clients and teaching workshops with a holistic approach to wellness, explaining why we, as a society, should stop fixating on remedying the by-products of poor nutrition and lifestyle choices through gimmicky, ineffective diets, and instead put that effort and money into correcting actual nutritional deficiencies.

I eventually realized that to truly address the health problems I was seeing, I needed to focus more attention on helping parents raise healthy children via proper nutrition. I was meeting way too many adults who refused to eat anything green (unless it was buried in cheese sauce), or raw, or made with whole wheat flour, and who, intentionally or not, were raising their kids to be the same way. The sad fact is that in the U.S., seven of the top ten leading causes of death, including coronary heart disease, diabetes, stroke, and various forms of cancer, are directly linked to diet and lifestyle. We live in one of the wealthiest countries in the world, we have some of the best doctors, we have modern medicines and hospitals, but we also have some of the highest

rates of chronic degenerative diseases in the world. Children are now being diagnosed with Type 2 diabetes, which used to be an illness associated mainly with adults.

I have seen firsthand the positive impact even simple dietary adjustments can have on one's health. I carry in my heart the story of a mama who came to one of my workshops. She was distraught: "My baby daughter has this ear infection that never seems to go away," she explained. "Her pediatrician is planning on putting in a tube since nothing seems to work. Is there anything else that can be done?" I asked if she would be willing to make some changes to what her baby was currently eating for at least a few weeks. "I will do anything, anything!" she replied.

So, we got to work. As a full-time working mother like me, she needed a manageable plan that didn't require her to cook food specifically for her baby every day. I came up with nutrient-dense batch recipes that she could multiply and freeze. We took out the baby cereals and replaced them with homemade purees including blueberry, banana, peas, butternut squash, sweet potato, lentils, avocado-mango, quinoa, and apple—all meals that are chock-full of antioxidants and also freeze well.

At the next workshop, the mama came in and excitedly told me that for the first time in three months her baby had gone three weeks without an earache or runny nose. "How come nobody ever mentioned that [the issue] might be her immune system due to nutritional deficiencies?" she cried. That is just one of hundreds of examples of clients of all ages whom I have helped.

Two years ago I spoke at the Comvita longevity panel at Expo West with Alan Bougen, the cofounder of Comvita; Dr. Mary Pardee, a functional medicine practitioner specializing in gut-brain health; and David Stewart, the CEO and founder of AGEIST. I shared the food philosophy I had learned from my mother, which came from rich, indigenous wisdom passed down from my grandmother and earlier generations of women, wisdom that science is finally recognizing as truth:

- Eat whole foods from the ground.
- Eat more whole plants.
- If you eat meat, let it be good-quality meat that was humanely pasture-raised.
- Seafood should be wild-caught.
- Don't eat too much meat or fish because a little goes a long way.
- Eat lots of fruit when it is in season.
- Most importantly, eat with gratitude, not guilt, and remember not to be greedy.

I want you to close your eyes as you hold this book in your hands and understand that it is yours to create magic, to reinvent yourself in the kitchen in ways you never thought possible. It doesn't matter if you weren't raised in a home with skilled cooks or entrenched in healthy food traditions as I was. It doesn't matter if you have no culinary experience at all. I am sharing my kitchen, my mami's kitchen, my grandma's bare-bones, gadget-free kitchen that produced the healthiest, most mouthwatering meals.

The title of this book, *Bountiful Cooking: Wholesome Everyday Meals to Nourish You and Your Family*, says it all. It is my life's purpose, what I want for my community, for each and every human on planet Earth regardless of age, background, or where they live: to grow and thrive without the daily headaches (and expense) of chronic, preventable diseases; to live a life bursting with vibrant energy; to age gracefully. We are always growing, from the day we are born to the day we die. It is never too late to start eating food and making lifestyle choices that will nourish your mind and your body. So long as there is breath in your body, you have the propensity for growth. This book you are holding—full of recipes, knowledge, life stories, and tips I share with my own family and clients—is an extension of who I am. I hope it helps and brings you joy, too.

Before you cook a single recipe, I encourage you to read this book from cover to cover. Not only can you then see the full range of ingredients and techniques used in the recipes, but you'll also glean lots of helpful information about how to deal with picky eaters, what produce is in season, what cookware you might need to replace, and much more. Above all, I hope this book leaves you with a sense of purpose and the confidence to take control of the health and well-being of you and your loved ones one meal at a time.

GETTING STARTED IN THE KITCHEN

You don't need to be a seasoned chef to cook for your family. What you need is nine out of ten parts affection and one part knowledge. Perfection is overrated. Cooking is about creating incredible memories, learning about different cultures, showing love in the most nurturing way, and even messing up. (Rest assured, that happens to the best of us and is a part of the process that needs to be cherished as well!)

Cooking good food at home is inextricably intertwined with good health, and this book is going to help you achieve and maintain the highest level of health for you and your family—and, I hope, do so from a place of joy. These recipes will nourish both your body and your soul. They are the same ones I cook in my home, share with my clients, and teach at workshops. As a full-time working parent juggling my own business with little free time, I am very conscientious about keeping my recipes almost absurdly straightforward, using ingredients you can generally find at your local grocery store. My goal is to get you in the comfort zone quickly so you can start cooking more intuitively, making changes here and there according to your (and your family's) preferences.

I know there are many factors that influence what we cook and how we eat, including religion, cost, culture, health goals, and allergies, but I truly believe there is something for everyone in this book. The recipes are flexible. Some of the meat and seafood dishes can be made vegetarian, and many of the vegetarian dishes can easily be adapted to vegan or by adding meat or fish. There are gluten-free and dairy-free recipes (and the latter will also work fine if you substitute with cow's milk). Feel free to leave out ingredients you don't like, replace them with ones you do, and mix and match mains and sides however you choose. I offer some of my favorite tips and practices below.

WE ARE WHAT WE EAT

One of the greatest gifts you can give to yourself, your family, and any other human you care about is robust health. And that starts with the deep, unshakable belief that everyday choices have the potential to impact health, especially when it relates to some chronic diseases, including diabetes, heart disease, and some cancers. From my observations as a health-care professional, a lot of us have not been raised to think we have any power over our health.

Multiple times a day we all make dietary and lifestyle choices that can either support our health or encourage disease. One of my favorite quotes is by the Australian actor and author F. M. Alexander, who said: "People do not decide their futures, they decide their habits and their habits decide their futures." While there are many factors that impact health, diet and nutrition are fundamental.

The Standard American Diet (SAD) contains too many unhealthy ingredients. A typical day for a family with kids may start with sugary cereal or pancakes or waffles made with refined bleached flour that is practically devoid of nutrients. Lunch is often a sandwich on bread made with refined bleached flour and cold cuts, and dinner is frequently pasta made with—you guessed it—refined bleached flour. Manufacturers take advantage of time-constrained consumers and offer profit-driven (instead of driven by health and well-being) convenience foods that are filled with artificial flavors and colors, high-fructose corn syrup, chemicals, and other unhealthy additives and preservatives. Some of those products come with a whopping two-to-four-year shelf-life, including baby food.

Part of the problem is that big nonprofit organizations focused on health and well-being, including the Academy of Nutrition and Dietetics, are partnered with the same large companies that manufacture many of the products negatively impacting people's health. Among some of the biggest sponsors of these nonprofits are Conagra, Sara Lee, Abbott, Kellogg's, General Mills, the Sugar Association, and the National Dairy Council. In 2018 I attended FNCE, the national conference of food and nutrition experts, and was shocked to see companies like Coca-Cola, McDonald's, and Kraft all offering nutrition information. Another part of the problem is government policies and practices that help to lower the cost of unhealthy foods. Unhealthy foods are cheaper because a big chunk of our nation's subsidies goes toward corn, soybean, wheat, cotton, rice, peanut, and dairy, making production of these more lucrative for farmers than growing fruits and vegetables. This also affects meat production because corn has become the predominate food for cattle. Less than 10 percent of the United States Department of Agriculture (USDA) subsidies are spent on fruits and vegetables. We hear all day, "Eat your fruits and vegetables," yet they aren't heavily subsidized to make them more accessible and cheaper for everyone, as soybean, corn, and wheat are. (If you would like to learn more about our food policies please visit the Environmental Working Group's Farm Subsidy Database, https://farm.ewg.org/.)

It is such a vicious circle. Americans do not need another fad diet or more supplements or medications. We need to go back to basics—the basics my mami taught me: Eat a healthy, balanced, varied diet that is minimally processed, with more fiber-rich fruits and vegetables and a moderate addition of good-quality protein and whole grains, nuts, and seeds. These are all the ingredients you will find in the recipes I'm sharing with you here. Even just a few changes to your meals can improve how you feel.

Pay attention to gut health, because more than 70 percent of the immune system is in the gut, and the immune system plays a critical role in the body's ability to fight off disease. A compromised immune system makes you more susceptible to practically every type of illness, and is linked to things like constant sniffling, colds, ear infections, rashes, cavities, and lethargy. I can't stress this enough: restoring and maintaining gut health is best done nutritionally, not pharmacologically. Consuming probiotic and prebiotic foods is more effective than consuming probiotic and prebiotic supplements. Likewise, when it comes to meeting the recommended daily intake of specific vitamins or minerals—or overcoming related deficiencies—try to do so with foods that are naturally rich in those vitamins or minerals. For instance, if you have an iron deficiency, eat more iron-rich foods, such as dark, leafy greens, lentils, or beef or chicken liver.

Of course, it's not easy to remember which foods are naturally high in what and how they benefit you, so I've compiled the following lists. Though not exhaustive, they provide a baseline for some of the most common deficiencies. You can use them in tandem with my recipes—choose the ones that fit the needs of you and your family and incorporate them into your everyday meals.

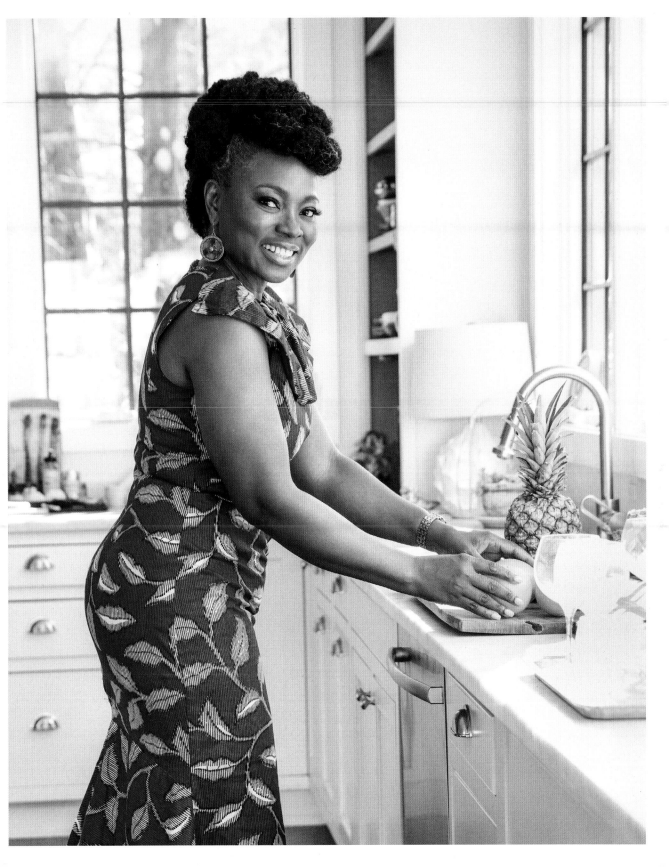

Important Nutrients, Benefits, and Food Sources

Probiotics

BENEFITS

Gut health. Probiotics are live microorganisms that have loads of health benefits for your mind, body, and spirit. They may help improve digestion, reduce depression, promote heart health, and reduce disease risk while also providing important vitamins, minerals, and protein. Because probiotics do not permanently stay in the intestinal tract, daily consumption of probiotics in some form is generally recommended.

FOOD SOURCES

Cassava, fermented

Corn, fermented

Kefir/Yogurt (preferably homemade; if using commercial, check the back label to verify that active or live cultures are listed; buy plain yogurt, and sweeten it at home to avoid unnecessary refined sugars)

Kimchi

Kombucha

Miso

Pickles (made with salt and water rather than vinegar; please read your labels if your pickles aren't homemade)

Sauerkraut

Tempeh

Prebiotics

BENEFITS

Gut health. Prebiotics are nondigestible nutritional compounds that are high in special types of fiber that support digestive health. These fibrous foods help maintain a healthy gut by increasing the presence and diversity of good bacteria. Prebiotics also help improve overall digestion and reduce the risk of leaky gut syndrome, candida, irritable bowl syndrome, and other intestinal issues. Prebiotics also help probiotics recolonize in the gut.

FOOD SOURCES

Apples

Cacao (nibs, powder, or bean)

Dandelion Greens

Dark Chocolate (80 percent cacao and above)

Flaxseed

Garlic

Jerusalem Artichokes

Jicama

Leeks

Lentils

Oats

Onions

Plantains

Seaweed

Soybeans

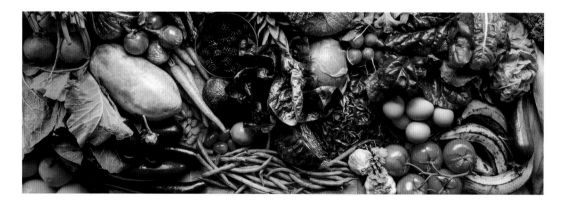

Polyphenols

BENEFITS

Polyphenols are compounds that we get through certain plant-based foods, and they're packed with antioxidants and potential health benefits. It's thought that polyphenols can improve or help treat digestion issues, weight-management difficulties, diabetes, neurodegenerative disease, and cardiovascular diseases.

FOOD SOURCES

Beans
Blueberries
Cherries
Cloves
Green Tea

Nuts (hazelnuts, walnuts, almonds, pecans)
Pomegranates
Soy

While I am not against vitamins and other supplements per se, I am opposed to having people think they are some kind of magic solution to their health woes. You can't eat junk food every day and then throw back a couple pills, powders, or potions and hope that all will be well. Supplements are supposed to support an already-healthy lifestyle, to give you an extra boost—hence the name. They cannot support what is not there. It's also important to note that this is a billion-dollar industry, and the motives of the companies involved can be more aligned with their pocketbooks than with your health.

Iron

BENEFITS

Iron is an essential nutrient during all stages of human development, but it's particularly important for children. The best way to improve iron levels is by eating foods that are high in iron.

FOOD SOURCES

FRUITS

Dates	Raisins
Figs	Unsulfured Dried Apricots
Prunes	

VEGETABLES

Broccoli	Potatoes
Brussels Sprouts	String Beans
Cabbage	Tomatoes
Dark, Leafy Greens (collards, kale, spinach)	

LEGUMES

Beans (black, cannellini, garbanzo, kidney)	Green Peas
	Lentils
	Soybeans

NUTS AND SEEDS

Almonds	Pine Nuts
Cashews	Pistachios
Flaxseed	Pumpkin Seeds
Hemp Seeds	Sesame Seeds
Macadamia Nuts	

MEAT AND SEAFOOD
(preferably pasture-raised/wild-caught)

Beef	Oysters
Chicken (and eggs)	Pork
Clams	Sardines
Haddock	Scallops
Lamb	Shrimp
Liver and Other Organs	Tuna
Mackerel	Turkey
	Veal

Calcium

BENEFITS

In addition to being an important building block for healthy bones and teeth, calcium is essential for every cell in the body. It serves as a signaling molecule and without it, your heart, muscles, and nerves would not be able to function.

FOOD SOURCES

FRUITS
Dried Figs

VEGETABLES
Bok Choy	mustard greens,
Dark, Leafy Greens (collards,	turnip greens, kale, spinach)

LEGUMES
Soybeans	Winged Beans
White Beans	

NUTS AND SEEDS
Celery Seeds	Poppy Seeds
Chia Seeds	Sesame Seeds

SEAFOOD
Salmon (canned, with bones, has a much higher percentage)	Sardines (with bones)

DAIRY
Cheddar Cheese	Plain Yogurt
Mozzarella Cheese	Ricotta Cheese

Magnesium

BENEFITS

Magnesium is essential for bone and tooth structure and helps boost energy, reduce inflammation, and support immunity, but many people do not consume the required daily intake. Low levels of magnesium are associated with several health conditions, including Type 2 diabetes, heart disease, and osteoporosis.

FOOD SOURCES

FRUITS
Avocados	Bananas

VEGETABLES
Dark, Leafy Greens	(collards, kale, spinach, swiss chard)

LEGUMES (dried suggested; canned as needed)
Black Beans	Peas (fresh or dried)
Chickpeas	
Lentils	Soybeans

NUTS AND SEEDS
Almonds	Chia Seeds
Brazil Nuts	Flaxseed
Cacao (nibs; powder; bean; dark chocolate, at least 80 percent cacao)	Peanuts (technically legumes, but most people consider them nuts)
Cashews	Pumpkin Seeds

WHOLE GRAINS
Barley	Quinoa (technically a seed, but most people use it as a grain)
Buckwheat	
Oats	
	Wheat

SEAFOOD (canned and fresh)
Halibut	(preferably wild-caught)
Mackerel	
Salmon	Tuna

Vitamin A

BENEFITS

Vitamin A is essential for overall health and well-being and supports immunity, reproduction, vision, the heart, lungs, kidneys, skin, and other organs, and cell growth. Insufficient consumption of it can lead to hair loss, skin problems, dry eyes, night blindness, and increased susceptibility to infections, among other conditions. As the human body cannot make vitamin A, you must obtain it from your diet or a supplement.

FOOD SOURCES

FRUITS

Cantaloupe	Pink and Red Grapefruit
Mangoes	

VEGETABLES

Broccoli	Red Bell Peppers
Carrots	Sweet Potatoes
Dark, Leafy Greens (collards, kale, turnip greens, spinach)	Winter Squash

LEGUMES

Black-Eyed Peas

MEAT

Beef Liver	Lamb Liver

SEAFOOD

Cod Liver Oil	King Mackerel
Herring	

Vitamin C

BENEFITS

Vitamin C is a potent antioxidant. It protects the body's cells and DNA from damage caused by free radicals, which can lead to cancer, and is vital for building and maintaining healthy bones, joints, skin, various tissues, and a strong immune system. It also helps your body absorb iron. While citrus fruits may be the most well-known and popular source of vitamin C, the items marked with an asterisk on the list below contain even higher amounts.

FOOD SOURCES

FRUITS

Black Currants	Papayas
Guavas*	Persimmons (American)
Kiwis*	
Lemons	Strawberries
Lychees	Tomatoes
Oranges	

VEGETABLES

Broccoli	Kale
Brussels Sprouts	Spinach
Chili Peppers	Snow Peas
Japanese Mustard Greens	Yellow Bell Peppers*

OTHER

Thyme (fresh)

Vitamin B$_{12}$

BENEFITS

Vitamin B$_{12}$ plays a vital role in healthy red blood cell formation, DNA synthesis, and the development and function of the brain and central nervous system. Vitamin B$_{12}$ deficiency may cause anemia with effects on cognitive development, as well as constipation, diarrhea, loss of appetite, vision impairment, irritability, depression, poor balance, muscle weakness, and numbness, among other things. In short, every cell in the body needs B$_{12}$ to function properly, but like most vitamins, the body can't produce it.

FOOD SOURCES

Beef

Dairy Products (preferably grass-fed/pasture-raised)

Eggs (preferably pasture-raised)

Organs (particularly kidneys and liver from lamb)

Seafood (particularly clams, sardines, tuna, trout, and salmon)

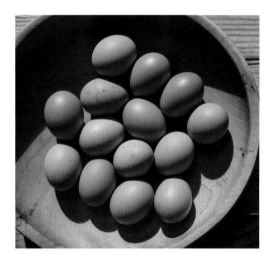

Fiber

BENEFITS

A fiber-rich diet helps promote ease and regularity of bowel movements and also helps to maintain a healthy weight by filling you up quickly and leaving you feeling full longer. Additionally, fiber lowers the risk of diabetes, heart disease, and some types of cancer, including colon and bowel cancer; encourages healthy gut bacteria; and cleans your colon.

FOOD SOURCES

FRUITS

Avocados

Apples (unpeeled)

Bananas

Blueberries

Guavas

Oranges

Pears

Prunes

Raspberries

Strawberries

Tomatoes

VEGETABLES

Artichokes

Beets

Broccoli

Brussels Sprouts

Carrots

Corn

Kale

Parsnips

Plantains

Potatoes (unpeeled)

Spinach

Turnip Greens

Winter Squash

LEGUMES

Beans (adzuki, black, kidney, lima, mung, and pinto)

Chickpeas

Lentils

Peas

Soybeans

NUTS AND SEEDS

Almonds

Chia Seeds

Pistachios

Pumpkin Seeds

Sunflower Seeds

Walnuts

WHOLE GRAINS*

Amaranth	Quinoa
Barley	Rye
Buckwheat	Sorghum
Bulgur	Teff
Corn	Wheat
Freekeh	Wild or Brown Rice
Millet	
Oats	

* Try to buy whole grain products such as breads, rolls, pancakes/waffles, baked goods, pasta, and the like whenever possible. And don't be fooled by the term "enriched grains." That means most of the fiber has been removed and a few vitamins added; the result is not nearly as healthy as the whole grain counterpart.

Vitamin D

BENEFITS

Vitamin D is critical in regulating the absorption of calcium and phosphorous and in facilitating immune-system health and the development of bones and teeth. Recent studies have also shown a connection between vitamin D deficiency in early pregnancy and language impairment and delayed mental and psychomotor development in the offspring's early childhood.

Unlike most vitamins—the body is capable of producing vitamin D, and all that's needed is exposure to direct sunlight. To maintain healthy blood levels, aim for ten to thirty minutes of midday sunlight, several times per week. People with darker skin may need a little more than this. Your exposure time should depend on how sensitive your skin is to sunlight.

FOOD SOURCES

Egg Yolks	Salmon
Herring	Sardines
Mushrooms	Shrimp

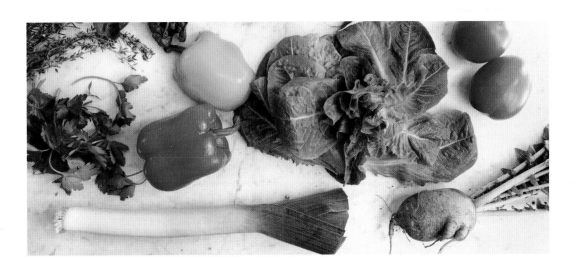

Folate

BENEFITS

Folate is important in the formation of healthy red blood cells, as well as cell growth and function. It is especially critical during periods of rapid growth, such as during pregnancy when the fetus is developing. The vitamin also plays a key role in breaking down homocysteine, an amino acid that can exert harmful effects in the body, such as contributing to dementia, heart disease, and stroke, if it is present in high amounts.

FOOD SOURCES

FRUITS

Bananas	Mangoes
Grapefruit	Oranges
Lemons	Papayas
Limes	

VEGETABLES

Arugula	Corn
Asparagus	Dark, Leafy Greens (kale, spinach, mustard, turnip)
Beets	
Broccoli	
Brussels Sprouts	Lettuce

LEGUMES

Black Beans	Lentils
Black-Eyed Peas	Peas (fresh and dried)
Chickpeas	
Kidney Beans	Soybeans

NUTS AND SEEDS

Almonds	Sunflower Seeds
Peanuts	

OTHER

Beef Liver	Wheat Germ
Eggs	

Zinc

BENEFITS

Zinc is an essential trace mineral that plays a role in more than a hundred enzymatic reactions in the human body. It helps with wound healing, blood clotting, immunity, metabolism, growth, and the ability to taste and smell.

FOOD SOURCES

LEGUMES*

Beans (adzuki, black, kidney, black-eyed peas)	Chickpeas
	Lentils

NUTS AND SEEDS

Almonds	Pine Nuts
Cashews	Pumpkin Seeds
Hemp Seeds	Sesame Seeds
Peanuts	Squash Seeds

MEAT

Beef	Lamb
Chicken	Pork

SEAFOOD

Crab	Mussels
Oysters	Shrimp

OTHER

Dairy Products	Tofu
Shiitake Mushrooms	

*Legumes contain high amounts of zinc, but they also contain phytates, which reduce the absorption of the mineral. Sprouting, soaking, or fermenting the legumes prior to cooking can help improve zinc's bioavailability.)

EAT THE RAINBOW

Red, orange, yellow, green, blue, purple, white, tan, and brown are all colors of the food rainbow, and each one contains phytonutrients with specific health functions and an abundance of nutrients with enormous healing powers. Eating a rainbow of colors in the form of fruits and vegetables each day is a fundamental key to sustainable health, ensuring your body gets a complete range of the vitamins and minerals needed to thrive. And the greater the variety of fruits and vegetables, the better. Ideally, you should incorporate three to five different colors of fruits and vegetables into your diet each week, but if that's not possible, do the best you can. (In case you are wondering, artificially dyed foods don't count and are, in fact, bad for you). To help get you going, here's a simple breakdown of each color, the fruits and vegetables that fall under it, and the primary related health benefits:

Red

PROTECTS HEART, LUNGS, AND PROSTATE

Red fruits and vegetables contain phytochemicals, including lycopene, ellagic acid, and a flavonoid called kaempferol. Those can be cancer-protective and can also help reduce the risk of heart disease. A high intake of lycopene, in particular, has been linked to a reduced risk of prostate cancer.

FOOD SOURCES

FRUITS

Blood Oranges	Raspberries
Cherries	Red Apples
Cranberries	Red Grapes
Pink/Red Grapefruit	Red Pears
	Strawberries
Pomegranates	Watermelon

VEGETABLES

Radicchio	Red Potatoes
Red Beets	Rhubarb
Red Onions	Tomatoes
Red Peppers	

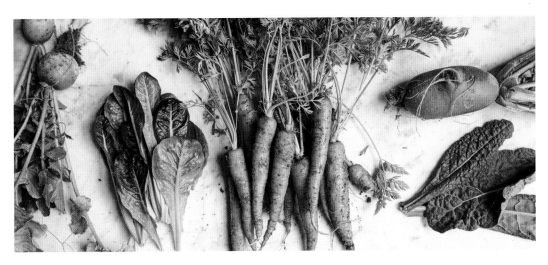

Orange and Yellow

PROMOTE EYE HEALTH

Phytochemicals known as carotenoids (beta-carotene, lutein, and zeaxanthin) give this group its bright colors. Lutein gets stored in the eye and has been shown to help protect against two of the most common causes of blindness: cataracts and age-related macular degeneration.

FOOD SOURCES

FRUITS

Apricots	Papayas
Cantaloupe	Peaches
Cape Gooseberries	Persimmons
Golden Kiwis	Pineapples
Grapefruit	Tangerines
Lemons	Yellow Apples
Mangoes	Yellow Figs
Nectarines	Yellow Pears
Oranges	Yellow Watermelons

VEGETABLES

Butternut Squash	Yellow Peppers
Carrots	Yellow Potatoes
Corn	Yellow Summer Squash
Pumpkins	Yellow Tomatoes
Rutabagas	Yellow Winter Squash
Sweet Potatoes	
Yellow Beets	

Green

PROTECTS AGAINST CANCER

Phytochemicals in green fruits and vegetables include varying amounts of flavonoids and carotenoids (beta-carotene, lutein, and zeaxanthin). The brassica group (broccoli, cabbage, and Brussels sprouts) also contains indoles, which can help to protect against cancer. Saponins, which are another powerful phytochemical found in green food plants, also have anticancer properties and may stop cancer cells from multiplying. Leafy greens are also an excellent source of folate (page 16).

FOOD SOURCES

FRUITS

Avocados	Honeydew Melons
Green Apples	Kiwis
Green Grapes	Limes
Green Pears	

VEGETABLES

Artichokes	Green Onions
Arugula	Green Peppers
Asparagus	Leeks
Broccoflower	Lettuce
Broccoli	Napa Cabbage
Broccoli Rabe	Okra
Brussels Sprouts	Peas
Celery	Snow Peas
Chayote Squash	Spinach
Cucumbers	Sugar Snap Peas
Endive	Watercress
Green Beans	Zucchini
Green Cabbage	

Blue and Purple

PROTECT AGAINST EFFECTS OF AGING

Blue and purple fruits and vegetables contain a group of phytochemicals known as flavonoids and anthocyanins, which have a mild antibacterial effect and are believed to delay cellular decay and help the heart by blocking the formation of blood clots. Resveratrol, which is most commonly found in grapes, may have a cancer-protective effect.

FOOD SOURCES

FRUITS

Blackberries	Plums
Black Currants	Purple Figs
Blueberries	Purple Grapes
Concord Grapes	Raisins
Elderberries	
Grape Juice (100 percent)	

VEGETABLES

Black Olives	(also known as red cabbage)
Black Salsify	
Eggplant	Purple Carrots
Purple Asparagus	Purple Peppers
Purple Belgian Endive	Purple Potatoes
Purple Cabbage	

White, Tan, and Brown

PROMOTE HEART HEALTH, STRONG BONES, AND GOOD CHOLESTEROL LEVELS

There are a lot of misconceptions about white food. I know you hear time and again to avoid it, but we're not talking about refined grains, sugar, bleached flour, or pasta here. Within the food rainbow, white (and tan and brown) encompasses potatoes, cauliflower, garlic, and the like. These foods are not as aesthetically vibrant as their colorful cousins, but they pack a powerful nutrition punch, for example, garlic and onion are chock-full of allicin and quercetin, powerful heart-promoting compounds; cauliflower is rich in sulforaphane, an anticancer compound; white button mushrooms are full of phytonutrients that have been found to inhibit aromatase activity and breast cancer cell proliferation. The next time you see a white whole food, ignore the voice telling you all white foods are bad.

FOOD SOURCES

FRUITS

Bananas	White Nectarines
Brown Pears	
Dates	White Peaches

VEGETABLES

Cauliflower	Mushrooms
Garlic	Onions
Ginger	Parsnips
Jerusalem Artichokes	Potatoes
Jicama	Shallots
Kohlrabi	Turnips
	White Corn

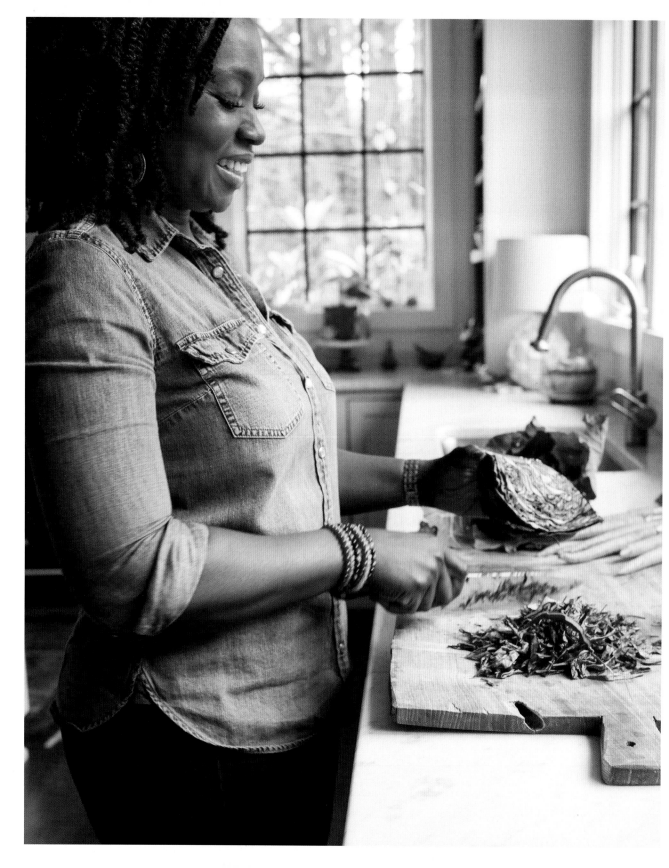

FOLLOW THE SEASONS

It can be hard to think of fruits and vegetables as seasonal nowadays, when you can get pretty much whatever you want whenever you want it at the supermarket or online. But it's important to realize that there are real benefits to eating seasonally, including:

MORE NUTRIENTS: In order for some fruits and vegetables to be available year-round, they are usually harvested before they are fully mature and postharvest treatments known as ripening agents are used before they hit the shelves. These include chemical, gas, and heat processes, and while these are all great for long-term storage, they can reduce nutritional value.

BETTER TASTE: Farmers who mass-produce fruits and vegetables year-round usually prioritize volume, appearance, and shelf life over taste, since the items need to travel across the country or the world. By contrast, smaller-scale farmers who grow produce as nature intended for a mostly local clientele don't need to rely on varieties of fruits and vegetables bred for sturdiness and can pick their crops at peak ripeness, or much closer to it than year-round producers can.

LOWER PRICES: Produce is abundant when it is in season and therefore is often much cheaper than at other times of the year. If you have access to a farmers market, you may find lower prices for fresh, seasonal produce by buying directly from the growers.

REDUCED CARBON FOOTPRINT: Out-of-season produce is typically shipped thousands of miles, which involves the burning of a lot of fossil fuel, which releases carbon dioxide into the air. If we all ate more local, in-season produce, that would have a big positive impact on the environment.

DECREASED PESTICIDE AND PRESERVATIVE CONSUMPTION: Out-of-season produce is usually subjected to a variety of pesticides and preservatives to maximize freshness and quality throughout its journey from farm to faraway store. Proper cleaning can remove some of those chemicals from the surface, but it's impossible to remove them all.

SEASONALITY MATTERS FOR MEAT AND FISH, TOO: You might also be surprised to hear that meat and some types of seafood have seasons, too. There's a reason turkey is traditionally served at Thanksgiving and ham at Easter. Beef, lamb, chicken, pork, and game are each at their best in terms of taste and texture at certain times of the year based on seasonal changes, migrations, environmental cues, and other factors. The same is true for some types of fish and shellfish.

To help you figure out what is best when, I compiled the following chart of the most popular foods to help guide you. But I also encourage you to dig deeper into what produce, meat, and/or seafood is available in your specific area from season to season, or in the case of something fleeting, like ramps or figs, for even shorter periods.

PRODUCE, SEAFOOD, AND MEAT BY THE SEASONS

	WINTER	SPRING	SUMMER	FALL
PRODUCE				
Apples	×	×	×	×
Apricots	×	×	×	
Artichokes				×
Arugula				×
Asparagus		×		
Avocados	×	×	×	
Bananas	×	×	×	×
Beets	×		×	×
Bell peppers			×	×
Blackberries			×	
Blueberries			×	
Broccoli		×		×
Brussels sprouts	×			×
Cabbage	×	×		×
Cantaloupe			×	×
Carrots	×	×	×	×
Cauliflower				×
Celery	×	×	×	×
Chard				×
Cherries			×	
Clementines	×			×
Collards	×	×		×
Corn			×	×
Cranberries				×
Cucumber			×	
Eggplant			×	×
Fennel				×
Garlic		×	×	×
Ginger				×
Grapefruit	×			
Grapes				×

	WINTER	SPRING	SUMMER	FALL
Green beans			×	×
Herbs	×	×	×	×
Honeydew melons			×	
Kale	×	×		×
Kiwi	×	×		×
Leeks	×			
Lemons	×	×	×	×
Lettuce		×		×
Lima beans			×	
Limes	×	×	×	×
Mangoes			×	×
Mushrooms		×		×
Okra			×	×
Onions		×		
Oranges	×			
Parsnips	×			×
Peaches			×	
Pears	×			×
Peas		×		×
Pineapples	×	×		×
Plums			×	
Potatoes	×			×
Pumpkins	×			×
Radishes		×		×
Raspberries			×	×
Rhubarb		×		
Rutabagas	×			×
Spinach	×	×		×
Strawberries			×	
Summer squash (yellow squash, zucchini)			×	
Sweet potato	×			×

	WINTER	SPRING	SUMMER	FALL
Swiss chard	×	×		
Tomatillos			×	
Tomatoes			×	×
Turnips	×	×		×
Watermelons			×	
Winter squash (butternut, acorn, spaghetti, kabocha, delicata, etc.)	×			
Yams	×			×
SEAFOOD				
Crabs		×	×	×
Haddock	×		×	×
Lobsters	×			×
Mackerel		×	×	×
Mussels	×	×		×
Oysters	×	×		×
Pacific salmon		×	×	×
Pollack	×	×	×	×
Prawns			×	×
Sardines		×	×	×
Scallops	×		×	×
Soft-shell crabs		×	×	
Tuna		×	×	×
MEAT				
Beef	×			×
Chicken		×		
Duck	×			×
Goose	×			×
Ham	×			
Lamb		×	×	×
Pork				×
Rabbit	×	×	×	×
Turkey	×	×		×
Venison	×		×	×

PANTRY STAPLES

"Agatha, where do I start? It is just so daunting." That is perhaps the question I am asked the most—at workshops, on social media, at parties—about transitioning to healthier eating habits, whether for a single person or a family. And my answer is always the same: Throw away items that aren't good for you and stock up on items that are. Having a well-stocked pantry, which includes your cupboards, fridge, and freezer, is one of the best ways to set yourself up for success. It also reduces stress—you should be able to make at least a few meals solely from pantry ingredients—and saves time and money thanks to no more last-minute runs to the store or ordering takeout.

When cleaning out your pantry, I suggest you toss (or give away) anything that meets at least one of the following criteria:

1. It is expired (that may seem obvious, but you'd be surprised...).

2. It has been around for a year (chances are you won't use it anyway).

3. The label includes ingredients that you can't pronounce.

4. The product contains more than ten ingredients.

As for what to stock, use the following list of healthy foods as a guide. It is by no means exhaustive, nor should you feel you have to purchase everything on it. Buy what makes sense for you and your family's tastes, dietary needs, budget, and cooking style, keeping in mind that some or all of that may change over time.

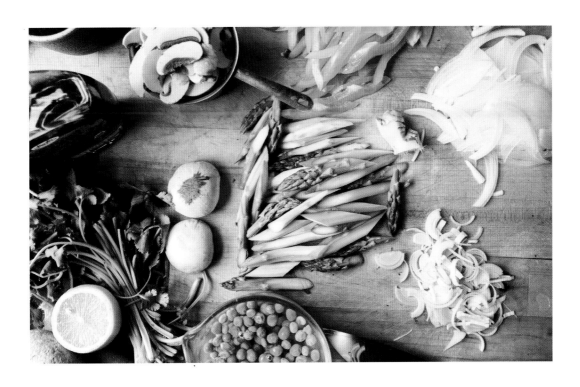

BOUNTIFUL EATING KITCHEN

Flours	Almond, brown rice, buckwheat, cassava, chickpea, coconut, corn, millet, oat, plantain, quinoa, spelt, teff, whole wheat flour (100 percent; nothing refined)
Whole grains	Amaranth, barley, buckwheat, bulgur, corn, farro, millet, quinoa, oats, brown rice, wheat
Dried legumes	Beans (adzuki, black, black-eyed peas, cannellini, fava, great Northern, kidney, mung, navy, pinto, red), chickpeas, lentils, peas
Nuts	Almonds, cashews, hazelnuts, macadamia nuts, peanuts, pecans, pine nuts, pistachios, walnuts
Seeds	Chia, flax, hemp, pumpkin, sesame, sunflower
Nut and seed butters	Almond, cashew, peanut, pecan, sunflower, tahini
Pasta	Brown rice, chickpea, lentil, potato, quinoa, whole wheat
Dried herbs and spices	Annatto, bay leaves, black cumin seed, black peppercorns, caraway seeds, cardamom, cayenne pepper, chili powder, cinnamon, coriander, crushed red pepper flakes, cumin, curry leaves, curry powder, fennel seeds, garlic powder, ginger, herbes de Provence, Italian seasoning, jerk seasoning, marjoram, mustard seeds, nutmeg, onion powder, oregano, parsley, rosemary, saffron, sage, sea salt, smoked paprika, sumac, tarragon, thyme, turmeric, za'atar
Dried fruits	Apricots, cranberries, cherries, mangoes, peaches, raisins (organic or sulfite-free; be aware that some processors use sulfites as a preservative, which can cause allergic reactions)
Canned items	Beans (black, red, white), broth (low-sodium), coconut milk, lentils (beluga black, brown, French green, green, red), olives, pasta sauce, salmon, sardines, tuna (wild-caught), tomatoes (diced, paste, pureed)
Oils/fats	Avocado oil, coconut oil, ghee, lard, nut oil (hazelnut, walnut, etc.), olive oil, extra-virgin olive oil, palm oil, sesame oil
Vinegars	Apple cider, balsamic, distilled, red wine, rice, white wine
Refrigerator items	Better Than Bouillon (organic), Bragg Liquid Aminos, capers, cheese (various, of good quality, including Parmesan), chili-garlic sauce, Dijon mustard, eggs (pasture-raised), fermented veggies (pickles, sauerkraut), fresh herbs, hot pepper sauce, jam (with no added sugar), ketchup, mayonnaise, minced garlic, milk (organic whole milk, if you truly love it, or unsweetened homemade or store-bought nut milks), miso paste, longer-lasting produce (apples, beets, cabbage, citrus, etc.), salsa, tamari (low-sodium), tempeh, tofu, tortillas, Worcestershire sauce

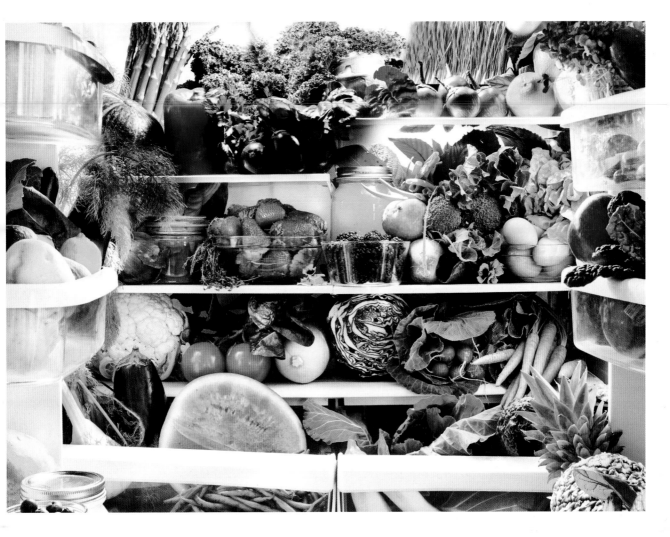

Freezer items	Bread, butter, cauliflower rice, cooked grains (rice, quinoa, oatmeal, etc.), fruit (blueberries, raspberries, bananas, etc.), meat, pancakes, sauces, seafood, soup, vegetables, veggie burgers, waffles
Longer-lasting produce	Acorn squash, butternut squash, cabbage, carrots, cassava, garlic, onions, plantains, potatoes, shallots, sweet potatoes
Sweeteners	Cane sugar, coconut sugar, date sugar, maple syrup (pure), monk fruit, raw honey, stevia
Tea	Your favorite herbal and green teas
Miscellaneous	Essentials you always need to have around. For me, that means arrowroot powder, aluminum-free baking powder, cacao powder, gluten-free baking soda, organic extracts (almond, peppermint, vanilla), nutritional yeast, vanilla beans, parchment paper, resealable plastic bags

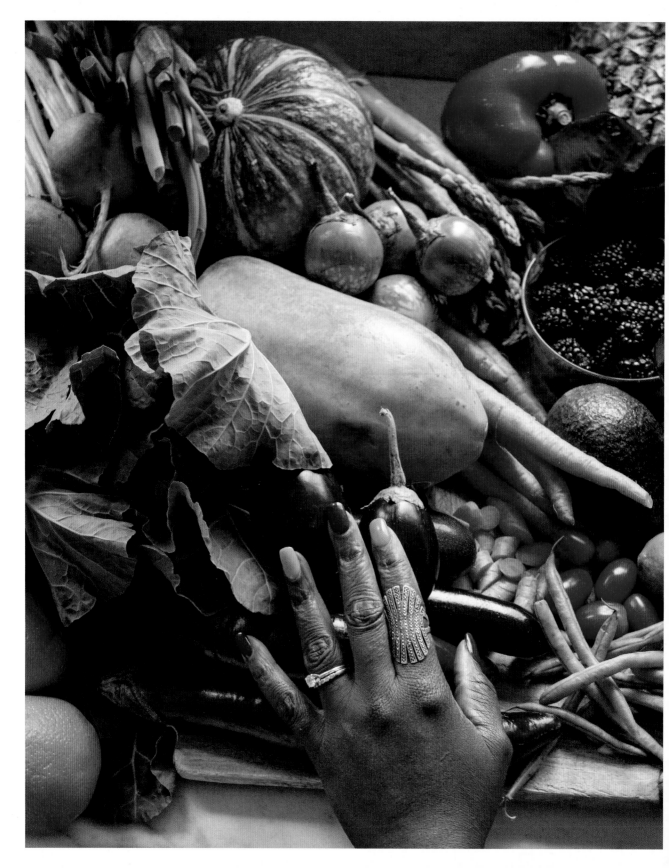

HEALTHY COOKWARE

We all have our favorite pots and pans, but I believe that you can't truly cook healthy food if you're using aluminum and coated nonstick cookware. Those materials are such a threat to our well-being, yet I cannot begin to tell you how many times I have watched someone on social media cooking a "healthy" recipe in a nonstick skillet, which allows toxins to be leached into the food. On the flip side, I've had clients and family members with chronic headaches get relief after replacing their coated and aluminum cookware.

For decades, a chemical named perfluorooctanoic acid (PFOA) was the standard material used to make nonstick cookware. After studies showed it was associated with various health problems, including liver tumors, breast cancer, reduced fertility, and thyroid and kidney disorders, it was banned in 2015. However, many people still own cookware that contains PFOA.

Polytetrafluoroethylene (PTFE)—a synthetic chemical commonly known as Teflon and formed by combining carbon and fluorine atoms—is now the primary coating used in nonstick cookware. It's very effective and very popular, but studies show that at temperatures above 570°F, it can start to break down, which can release toxic chemicals into the air. Inhaling those fumes can lead to flu-like symptoms, such as chills, fever, headache, and body aches. Even scarier, birds exposed to the fumes can die within seconds! Meanwhile, when you look at a peeling nonstick pan, ask yourself where those particles went.

As for the issues with aluminum cookware, food can react with the metal to form aluminum salts that have been associated with dementia, Alzheimer's disease, and impaired visual motor coordination. Indeed, research into that began when aluminum deposits were found in the brains of Alzheimer's sufferers during autopsies.

Before I get to the good news about better options, here is a tip I follow in my home and that I share with clients when faced with new or conflicting information about what is "safe" or not: Err on the side of caution. Prioritize your health and your family's health and understand that big companies often make decisions based on profit and loss, not people's health and well-being. Replacing some or even all of your cookware is a small price to pay when you consider the possible effects using aluminum or coated nonstick items may have on your health.

Cookware made from the following materials is free of PTFE, PFOA, and per- and polyfluoroalkyl substances (PFAS), and won't react with food the way aluminum can. And a well-seasoned, properly heated cast-iron pan, for instance, can be very effective when it comes to preventing food from sticking:

Stainless steel	Ceramic (lead-free)
Glass	
Terracotta (without a lead-based glaze)	Cast-iron

My Favorite Kitchen Equipment

Having a basic set of mixing bowls, measuring cups and spoons, and a cutting board are all good basics that you may already have. In addition, I have the following in my kitchen:

KNIVES: Listen, invest in a good-quality chef's knife; a good knife is the difference between night and day compared to the regular knives you see everywhere. A good knife is not cheap but worth every penny. I bought my first good-quality knife at thirty-five years of age and paid at the time an unbelievable $175, OMG. Don't wait too long the way I did. Trust me, you don't need nine different knives in your home kitchen; a chef's knife, a paring knife, and a serrated knife are the basics you need.

SHARPENING STONE: When you experience life with a good-quality, sharp chef's knife you will never want to cook with anything less. But you need to take care of your knife and that's where a sharping stone is a must-have. My husband, Georges, sharpens my knives regularly. I love him so for this.

POTATO RICER: This will give you the creamiest potato but also multitask as a baby food masher. With the kiddos grown, I still use this to quickly mash banana into oatmeal as a sweetener.

MANDOLINE SLICER: For French fries, the perfect cucumber and radish rounds, and finely shredded cabbage, a mandoline is a superstar.

MICROPLANE: Did you know that lemon zest contains fiber, calcium, potassium, and magnesium, and that consuming even small amounts is beneficial to your health? Lemon zest also enlivens countless sweet and savory foods, from pancakes to marinades to salad dressings. So, keep a microplane at the ready, and never throw a lemon rind in the trash without zesting it first! You can buy a microplane at the hardware store for as little as $3; it is also perfect for grating garlic, ginger, turmeric, and nutmeg.

SALAD SPINNER: Once you have a spinner, you can make your weekly salad at home instead of buying premade bags. A spinner makes quick work of drying herbs and leafy vegetables, which helps keep them fresh. The interior basket can double as a colander for cold foods.

SPICE GRINDER / COFFEE BEAN GRINDER: If you buy seeds, such as cumin, coriander, or flax, already ground, I suggest you invest in a spice grinder and grind them yourself. Compared to freshly ground seeds, preground ones are more expensive, aren't as potent, and go rancid faster. Grinding your own takes just a minute or so and is well worth it. You'll find your food tastes better, too!

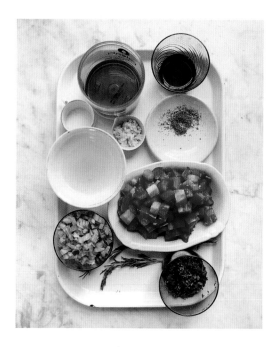

MAKE FRIENDS WITH
YOUR FREEZER

The freezer is an incredibly useful appliance, and highly underrated. For busy people, older kids, smaller families, or someone undergoing medical treatments, for example, the freezer can help ensure that a healthy, wholesome meal is always at the ready.

That said, some dishes freeze better than others. Generally speaking, soups, stews, pastas, casseroles, breaded cutlets, oatmeal, grains, and baked sweets are good candidates for freezing (in fact, I batch-cook things like brown rice, quinoa, and millet and freeze them in freezer-friendly reusable bags). I also freeze raw ingredients that are at risk of going bad. Avoid freezing items that contain a lot of watery ingredients, such as cabbage or zucchini, as well as cream sauces and eggs, as the texture really breaks down when thawing.

There are varying opinions on the best freezing methods, but these are the guidelines I follow and share with my clients. As always, do what works best for you.

FREEZING
BREADED CUTLETS

Whether chicken, pork, or veal, breaded cutlets freeze really well uncooked or cooked, so I usually make a big batch and set some aside for another meal or two. In order to ensure that the cutlets don't stick together, I separate them with small pieces of parchment paper before placing them in a large reusable freezer bag or container.

- For the best flavor, color, texture, and nutrient content, slightly undercook food that you plan to freeze and reheat.

- Allow cooked foods to cool completely before storing in the freezer, but cool them on the counter rather than in the fridge, to avoid raising the temperature in the refrigerator and causing other foods to spoil. (That said, the food should not sit at room temperature for longer than about two hours, depending on what it is and the temperature of the house.) If you're in a hurry, cool food in a container set in ice water that comes halfway up the sides.

- If you're freezing food for less than two months, regular plastic bags or wrap are adequate, as long as they have an airtight seal, to decrease the risk of freezer burn, which occurs when air meets frozen food. Freezer burn is not harmful, but it adversely affects the food's texture and color.

- If you're freezing food for longer periods, use heavy-duty aluminum foil lined with parchment paper, laminated freezer paper, plastic freezer bags, or freezer wrap. You can also use heavy-duty BPA-free plastic containers or freezer-safe glass containers. Remember to leave head space in containers, because foods expand during freezing; remove any excess air from bags before sealing. Whatever you use, the packaging should be airtight. This all makes a big difference in post-thaw quality.

- Freeze food in portions that make sense for you and your family. You don't want to have to defrost a container of stew that feeds eight when you're feeding only three.

- Properly label containers and packages with the name of the contents and the date they were prepared. Instructions for reheating are also helpful depending on who will be reheating the food.

- Thaw food in the refrigerator where it will remain at a safe, constant temperature of 40°F or below. That's also the gentlest method in terms of preserving the best texture and taste.

However, as a full-time working parent, I also know that life happens—I can't tell you how many times we would all get home and realize we forgot to move our dinner from the freezer into the refrigerator. If you are in a time crunch, you can place sealed food in a large bowl or pot filled with cold water that you change every thirty minutes until the food is thawed.

- For the best flavor and texture, frozen foods should be consumed within six to nine months.

- Lastly, if your budget permits and you freeze items frequently, consider investing in a vacuum sealer. It removes as much excess air as possible and saves space in the freezer. I don't have one, but some people swear by them.

FREEZING VEGETABLES

When that head of broccoli, bunch of carrots, or bag of string beans is about to go bad, rather than resign yourself to throwing it away, blanch and freeze the vegetables. It takes only a few minutes and then on another busy night when you want some veggies, all you need to do is pop them in boiling water, drain, and season (or use in another recipe). To blanch, first prep and cut the vegetables as desired, then place them in boiling water for about thirty seconds. Drain and quickly submerge them in ice water to prevent them from cooking further. When they are cold, drain them thoroughly, then place them in a freezer-friendly reusable bag or container and freeze them.

MEAL PLANNING

Meal planning is key to creating healthy, nutritious meals on a regular basis and can save you even when schedules seem to be spinning out of control. Although not every meal you cook has to be healthy, cooking is one of the best ways to support your health. There are many other benefits to meal planning, too. Here are my top four:

1. It saves time and money: Grocery shopping is more focused, there's less impulse buying, and there's less need for last-minute runs to the store. Planning ahead also helps limit the number of occasions you resort to takeout or fast food. Although at first, meal planning might feel time-consuming, once you do it a couple times, it will become much faster and easier and will ultimately reduce the time you spend thinking about and coming up with meals each week.

2. It provides more variety: When you sit down and plan your meals, you are more intentional about them and can create a thoughtfully composed and balanced menu that integrates new flavors, dishes, and even cuisines you've been wanting to try.

3. It is less stressful: It's incredibly freeing not to have to worry about what you're going to make for breakfast, lunch, and dinner every day! Even if you just plan a few meals a week, you will save yourself the anxiety that comes with thinking about what you are going to cook multiple times a day.

4. It prevents food waste: Meal planning promotes more conscientious grocery shopping and helps you pay better attention to a food's shelf life. When you plan ahead and shop from a list, you are also less likely to buy extra food that may go bad before you can eat it.

Getting Started

While there is no perfect, one-size-fits-all approach to meal planning, over the years, I've come up with a list of suggestions that you may find helpful as you get started.

- Don't be too ambitious. Meal planning only works if you actually stick to your plan, so keep it simple, at least at the beginning or when you know you have an especially busy week ahead. If you are new to meal planning, I recommend planning only one week at a time. When you are comfortable with that and want to do more, you can try biweekly or monthly planning. We all have different lifestyles, so experiment and find what works best for you and your family.

- Keep breakfast and lunches basic and repetitive. Unless you're someone who already cooks breakfast and lunch every day, cooking three meals a day is going to be way too much. You can still plan those meals, as well as snacks and treats—and I highly recommend you do so to avoid more trips to the store or resorting to takeout or unhealthy meals. Just be sure your planned meals are manageable and involve minimal or batch cooking. For instance, scale up my Quinoa Waffles (page 57) and serve them for breakfast several times that week.

- Let each family member select at least one meal they would love to eat each week. (For birthdays and other special occasions, it's also fun to let the honoree pick the entire week of meals.) That system has worked really well in my house—everyone is more invested in what we eat, and it has even brought us closer. Of course, the cook has the final say and can balance the selection in terms of variety, dietary needs, workload, schedule, cost, and so on.

- Include a few multifunctional—or, as I call them, all-purpose—recipes in the mix to save time and effort. For example, a big batch of black bean stew can be eaten with rice one day, added to a burrito the next day, and tossed with greens, whole grains, and store-bought salsa another day.

- Write it down. Technology has made this so easy with apps and electronic reminders, but I am old school and still write my weekly menus and the accompanying shopping list in a notebook.

- Consider planning and shopping on one day and prepping (washing lettuces, chopping vegetables, making a large pot of grains, cooking a couple of main courses to be reheated later in the week) on another. I find that less hectic than doing everything on the same day. However, whatever works best for you is the best way.

- Be flexible and remember always to give yourself grace. Life will happen—kids' activities run late, you're stuck in a meeting, the dog gets sick, you forget to defrost the ground beef. Don't hesitate to rejigger the menu, and if all else fails and you have to order a pizza, that's totally okay.

- Have a backup plan. In order to avoid having to call for that pizza, keep a few pantry/freezer meals at the ready that you or someone else, even a teen, can get onto the table quickly and easily.

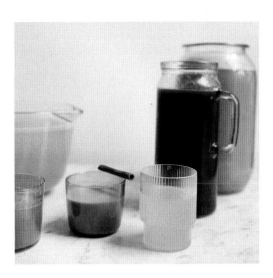

PICKY EATERS— KIDS AND ADULTS!

What I love so much about the human body is its capacity to heal when provided the nourishment it needs—there is always an upside to changing unhealthy habits. However, the earlier you start, the better, which is why it is particularly important for parents to do what they can to feed their kids wholesome, nutritious food and limit sugary drinks and snacks loaded with artificial ingredients. That will help set them up for a lifetime of good choices at the grocery store and the table while optimizing their general health. What happens, though, when one or more of your kids is a so-called picky eater?

> "My kid won't touch anything green. All he'll eat is cereal."

> "My child likes chicken nuggets, French fries, and macaroni and cheese. That's it."

> "My son will only taste the green stuff on the plate if he gets a cookie afterward."

> "Vegetables? Potatoes are a vegetable, right?"

> "At Thanksgiving, she ate five dinner rolls. We couldn't get her to touch anything else."

> "My son screams at the sight of vegetables. He won't stop until he gets what he wants."

Those are actual quotes I've heard from parents over the years. I get it! It's really hard to fight battles around food, especially when you have so much else going on. But those are battles parents must win because children cannot thrive without proper nutrition. Many common childhood ailments, including asthma, ear infections, attention-deficit hyperactivity disorder (ADHD), allergies, Type 2 diabetes, and constipation, are linked to diet. Furthermore, studies have shown that many of the short- and long-term health issues adults face can be traced back to dietary issues stemming from their childhood.

Until I moved to the States, I had never heard about picky eating. Back home, kids ate whatever was placed in front of them. So, I was surprised the first time a client told me her eighteen-month-old daughter wouldn't eat green vegetables. "I just can't make her try anything green," she lamented. "She cries and throws up." Well, it took us almost seven months of smoothies, vegetable-infused muffins, steamed vegetables, and green juices to get that child to willingly eat green food. We would offer it almost every day and every day she would turn it down, sometimes after a tiny bite or a sip or two. My spinach, mango, and pineapple smoothie eventually did the trick. She loves mangoes, and this time she sat watching as the smoothie was made, asking for a piece of juicy mango. She took a sip, this time around she didn't stop. I'm happy to report that she is now a young mother of two amazing girls, who also love their greens.

After meeting other families, friends, and clients with picky eaters of all ages, I was eager to learn how food aversions begin, as well as more ways to help parents solve this issue with less frustration. A study by Betty Ruth Carruth, PhD, RD; Paula J. Ziegler, PhD, RD; Anne Gordon, PhD; and Susan I. Barr, PhD, RDN, published in the January 2004 issue of the *Journal of the American Dietetic Association* revealed that parents typically offered their infants and toddlers foods only once or twice before deciding whether they liked it. The conclusion was that parents gave up trying a little too soon and inadvertently encouraged their children to be picky.

Age is also a factor. Once children have started walking and beginning to speak, they develop a sense of independence and the consciousness to act upon it. Whether they like a particular food or not, they can refuse to open their mouth, run away, cry in protest, throw a tantrum or, as many of us know, do all of the above. Along with increased independence, a child begins to notice a pattern: There are foods that are sweet and foods that are not sweet, and of course the child would like the sweet food. Also complicating matters is that the vast majority of commercial baby foods combine vegetables with apples, bananas, or pears—sweeter fruits. A baby who has grown accustomed to eating such products develops a palate for sweet foods. If the parent then attempts to introduce an unsweetened green vegetable, the child usually notices the difference and refuses it.

Parents also tend to impose their own food preferences on children. For example, parents who do not like okra or brown rice do not cook those foods for themselves and therefore do not give them to their children (and this is where adult picky eaters come in!). It's important for parents to remember that eating is a learned behavior beginning with the very first spoonful, and is reinforced with each and every meal.

Check out my top tips for cultivating a child with a flexible palate and open mind when it comes to food. It can be difficult and time-consuming, but it is absolutely worth doing. Be patient, be consistent, and give yourself grace and your child will likely explore a wider range of foods. Note that adults can have these issues as well and while my tips are written for parents of picky eaters, they do apply to adults, too—we can all broaden our palate, no matter our age.

Don't stop trying to introduce new foods too soon. As mentioned earlier, many parents aren't aware of the lengthy, yet normal course of food acceptance in children. Touching, smelling, playing with, and spitting out food are all normal exploratory behaviors that can happen before acceptance—and some kids simply take longer to develop a taste or affinity for a food. Keep trying and be consistent. Remember, how you manage this will set the stage for pickiness going forward.

Don't be a short-order cook. Often, parents of multiple children will make a variety of dishes for a single meal in order to appease each child. That kind of short-order cooking is tiring and unsustainable, and only serves to entrench the problem you are trying to correct. There's no reason for any child to stop being picky if preferred options are always readily available. Unless a child has an allergy or sensory issue, such as a texture aversion, then they should be able to eat whatever you serve. It doesn't make you a bad mama to stand firm on that.

Don't make up for missed meals with junk food. If your child refuses to eat a meal because they don't like the options available, don't offer junk food just to fill their belly. Remember, your child needs you to help them make the right choices, even when they are adamant about what they want.

Don't force a clean plate. Even though you may be anxious about making sure your child is getting the necessary nutrients needed for growth and development, I don't recommend forcing them to eat every bite. That can actually make them even pickier! Your child is not trying to frustrate you. Again, food acceptance takes time. Also, forcing clean plates can cause a child to lose their natural sense of knowing when they are full, which can then lead to overeating and obesity. Building healthy eating habits means respecting when your child says they are full even when you think they haven't had enough.

Do expose your child to a wide variety of foods. Introduce your child to an array of flavors and textures no matter what your own personal preferences or aversions may be (and perhaps use this opportunity to try new foods yourself!). Your child may very well love the foods you dislike. Try new dishes, including foods from other parts of the globe, at least once a month, and for older kids, take the opportunity to tie the dish to its origins and make it a fun learning experience. I've also had success getting kids to eat an ingredient they don't like by adding it to a tried-and-true dish. For instance, stirring a cup of chopped fresh parsley into their favorite pasta (maybe on Italian night) might be the magic that changes their relationship with all things green.

Stock the foods you want your child to eat. Your child—and any adults—can only be as picky as the food options that are made available to them. If you no longer want your child to eat macaroni and cheese or French fries or cookies at home, don't buy them. You can't necessarily control everything they eat when they aren't with you, but you sure can at home. Filling your refrigerator and pantry with healthy, nutritious food options is the first step.

Treat every snack as an opportunity to nourish your child with good food. Instead of viewing snack time as "treat" time, think of it like a mini healthy meal and feed your child accordingly. (This book includes fifteen good-for-you snacks and treats, including Strawberry Chia Pudding (page 100) and

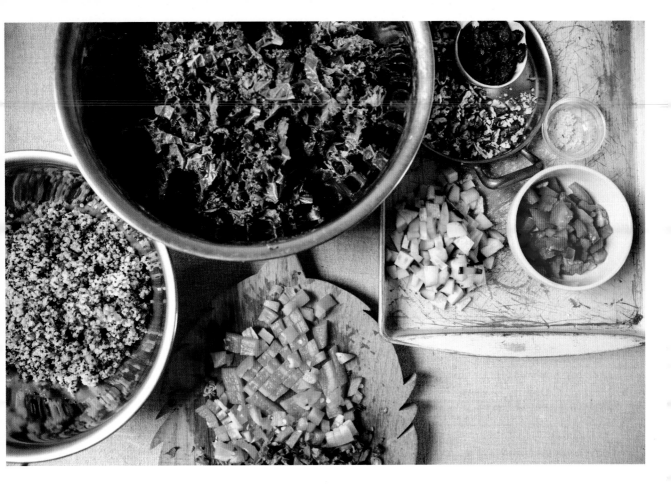

Baked Sweet Potato Doughnuts (page 119) that my family and clients both young and old enjoy.)

Involve your kids in the kitchen and make every eating experience pleasant. As many studies have shown, children who help with meal preparation are more likely to eat the resulting food, so let your child pitch in, and make cooking a family activity when possible. Spend an extra minute or two on presenting food in a visually appealing way; even kids eat with their eyes first. Lastly, be sure to take into account your child's texture preferences. For example, don't overcook string beans when they prefer them crisp.

Keep your children and yourself hydrated. Children—and adults—often prefer sugary drinks over water. Aside from the effects of consuming refined sugar, the problem is that a lot of the products sold in the ever-growing supermarket drinks aisle don't hydrate you; they actually do the opposite. And dehydration can lead to many problems, including headaches, constipation, excess body fat, fatigue, and heat injury. So, if your child is thirsty (as opposed to just wanting a special treat), please give them water. Bonus: water is readily available and generally free or relatively inexpensive compared to other beverages, so drink up!

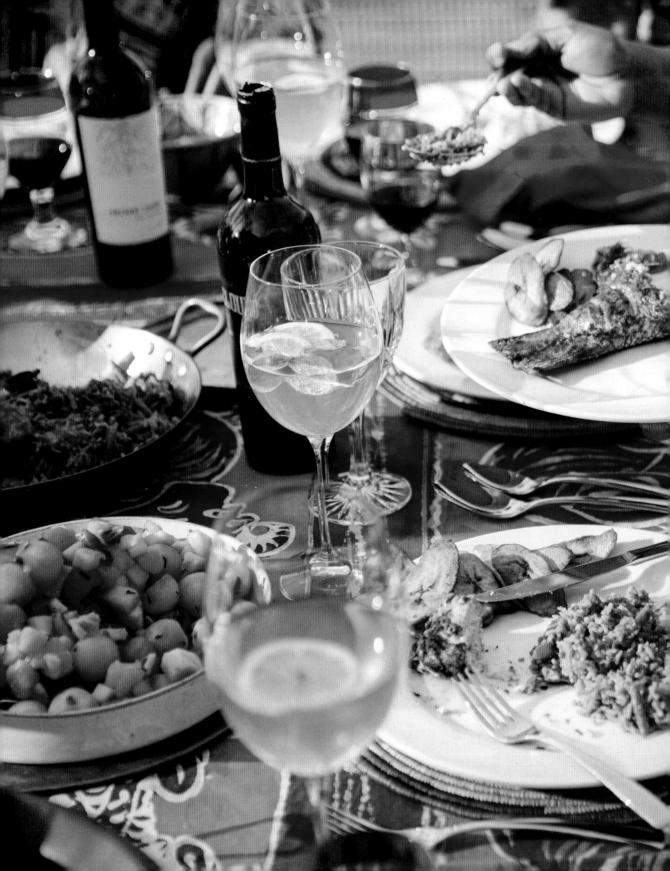

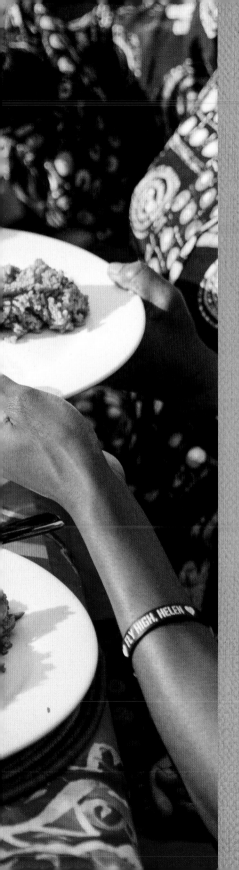

THE
RECIPES

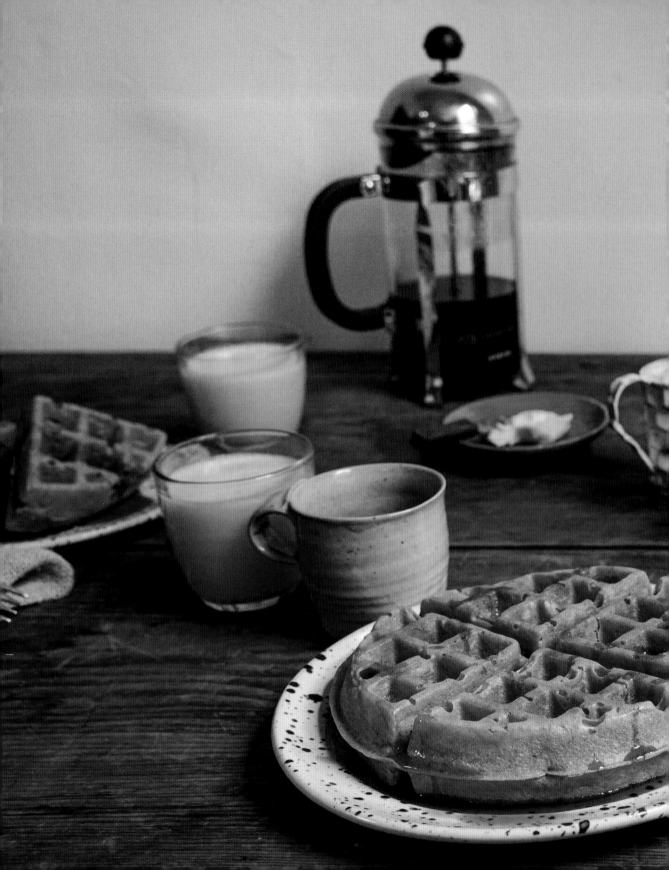

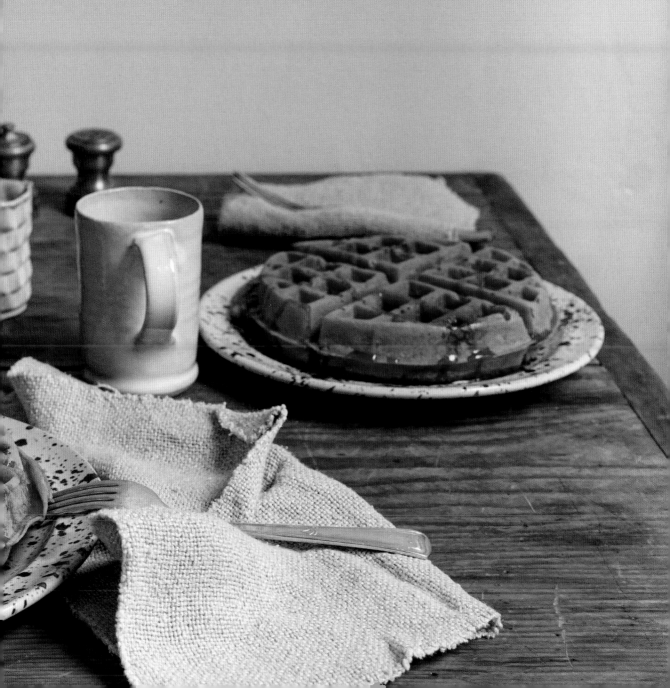

Breakfast

W<small>E'VE ALL HEARD THE MAXIM</small> "Breakfast is the most important meal of the day," and it exists for good reason. As the name suggests, breakfast is how we break our overnight fasting period. That meal should power you into your day and help your body perform at its best, by jump-starting your metabolism and replenishing your supply of natural glucose to boost energy levels and alertness, while also providing other essential nutrients required for good health.

However, eating the Standard American Diet (SAD) breakfast—that is, sugary and/or highly refined cereals, breakfast bars, pancakes, and waffles filled with synthetic ingredients— is one of the most unhealthy dietary habits in existence today and unfortunately this habit is slowly spreading across the globe. Such a breakfast lacks the vital nutrients the human body needs and instead is loaded with highly refined and synthetic ingredients with very few life-sustaining nutrients.

I know life is hectic and convenience is important, but don't underestimate the impact you can have on your health, and your family's health, by coming up with simple alternatives to that morning bowl of sugary cereal or highly refined pancakes or waffles. I did that myself, and trust me when I say there were lots of tears (from both the adults and the kids!), but it was so worth the effort.

A good place to start is the recipes in this section. Some are super quick, some are perfect when you are on the go, some are make-ahead, some are for a leisurely Sunday. But each and every recipe is both super tasty and super nutritious. Try my easy Granola recipe (page 44). I suggest scaling up the recipe; it's that good. Maybe serve it with one of my homemade milks (beginning on page 269), and enjoy a quick wholesome breakfast that will give you the same crunch and feel of cereal without the unnecessary ingredients. It's totally doable—I promise!

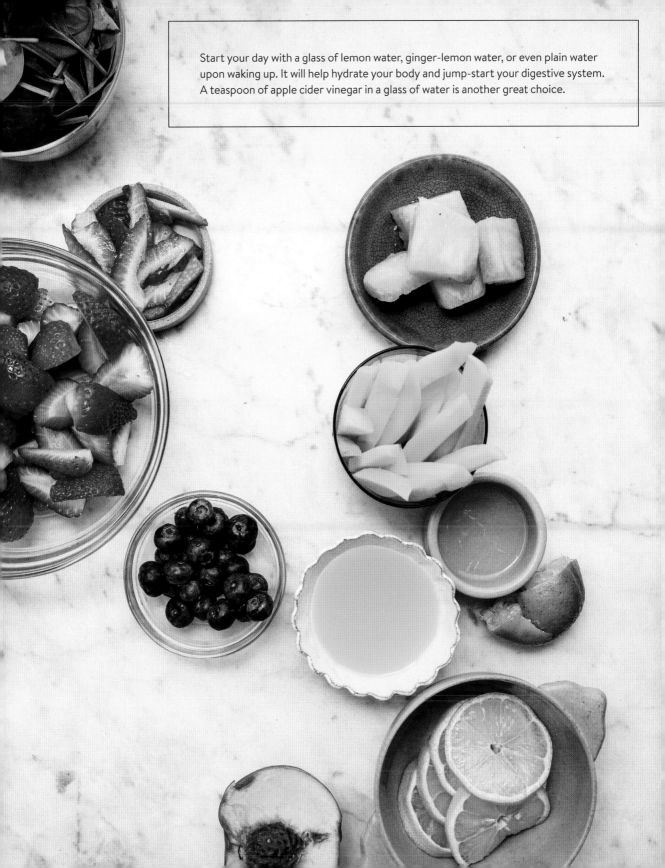

Start your day with a glass of lemon water, ginger-lemon water, or even plain water upon waking up. It will help hydrate your body and jump-start your digestive system. A teaspoon of apple cider vinegar in a glass of water is another great choice.

GLUTEN-FREE (GF)
DAIRY-FREE (DF)
SERVES 8

4 cups gluten-free
  sprouted oats
1 cup raw almonds
½ cup buckwheat
  groats
1 cup shredded
  coconut,
  unsweetened
1 cup dried cranberries
1 cup raw pecans,
  chopped
1 cup raw pumpkin
  seeds
2 teaspoons ground
  cinnamon
2 teaspoons sea salt
8 tablespoons coconut
  oil
½ cup maple syrup
2 teaspoons vanilla
  extract

Granola

On days you want to just pour a bowl of cereal for breakfast but still want to it to be super healthy and tasty, this granola is your answer. It's chock-full of immunity-boosting and gut-friendly fiber, antioxidants, minerals, essential vitamins, protein, and good fats, not to mention good carbs. It also keeps in the freezer for up to three months, so make a big batch! Healthy food can be comforting, nourishing, and healing.

Preheat the oven to 350°F and line a large rimmed baking sheet with parchment paper.

In a large mixing bowl, combine the oats, almonds, buckwheat groats, coconut, cranberries, pecans, pumpkin seeds, cinnamon, and salt. Stir to blend.

Pour in the oil, maple syrup, and vanilla. Mix until every ingredient is lightly coated. Pour the granola onto your prepared pan and use a large spoon to spread it in an even layer.

Bake until lightly golden, about 20 minutes, stirring halfway (for extra-clumpy granola, press the stirred granola down with a spatula to create a more even layer).

Let the granola cool completely, at least 45 minutes. Break the granola into pieces with your hands if you want big chunks, or stir it around with a spoon if you do not.

Store the granola in an airtight container at room temperature for 1 to 2 weeks or in a sealed freezer bag in the freezer for up to 3 months. Let it warm to room temperature for 5 to 10 minutes before serving.

Baked Oatmeal

Oatmeal is like a little black dress: There is no right or wrong way to wear it, but there is always a way to take it up a notch. Here, I take it up a notch by using sprouted oats, adding many amazing gut-healing nutrients, such as fiber, omega-3 fatty acids, and magnesium, and baking the mixture. It is so tasty and comforting. Please, do not use fast-cooking oats for this recipe. Please note, you can make this vegan by replacing the eggs with 4 tablespoons of ground flaxseed and an additional ½ cup of Almond Milk (page 269). You can eat the oatmeal as is or with your favorite toppings. (I like it with warm milk.)

Preheat the oven to 375°F. Grease a 13 × 9–inch baking pan or 12-inch cast-iron skillet with oil.

In a large bowl, mix together all the dry ingredients. In another large bowl, whisk together the eggs (or flaxseed and extra almond milk if making a vegan option), almond milk, and vanilla until the mixture is nice and frothy, then whisk in the melted coconut oil.

Pour the wet mixture over the dry mixture and stir well to combine into a porridge-like batter. Transfer the batter to the prepared baking sheet, spreading and flattening it evenly with a spatula.

Bake until the oatmeal achieves a pleasing golden-brown color on top and a knife inserted into the center comes out clean and free of liquid, 40 to 45 minutes. By that time, the fragrance of baked oats, dried fruit, nutmeg, and cinnamon will have perfumed your kitchen.

Let cool slightly before cutting.

¼ cup coconut oil, melted, plus more for greasing the skillet

3 cups sprouted gluten-free oats (or any type of rolled oats)

1 cup raw pecans, chopped

½ cup dried whole blueberries, preferably wild

½ cup dried cranberries

2 tablespoons hemp seeds

2 teaspoons baking powder

1 teaspoon ground cinnamon

1 teaspoon freshly grated nutmeg

6 large eggs, or 4 tablespoons ground flaxseed mixed with ½ cup Almond Milk (page 269)

2 cups Almond Milk (page 269) or whole milk

1 teaspoon vanilla extract

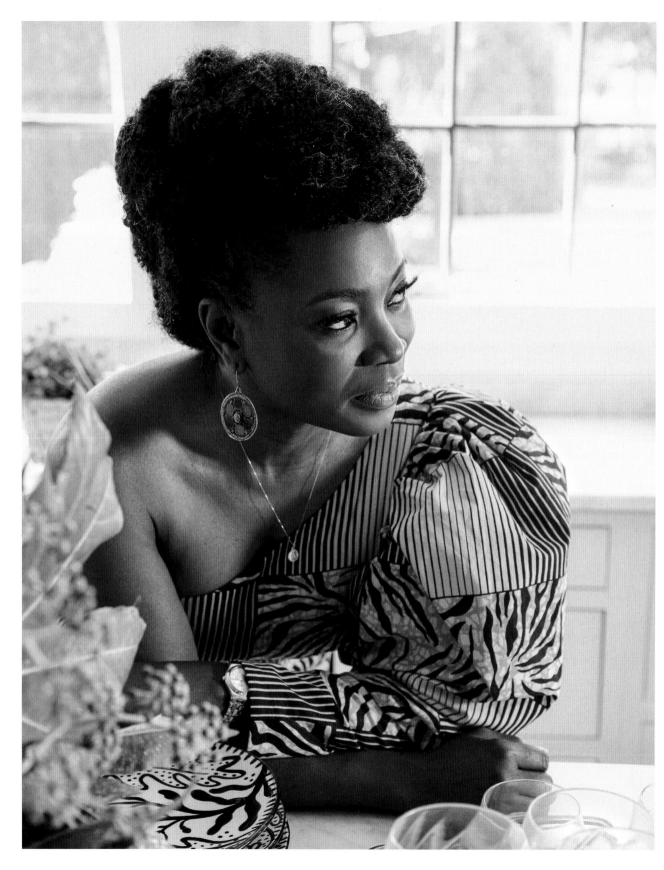

Egg- and Dairy-Free Blueberry Pancakes

1 cup very ripe mashed banana (it should be mostly smooth)

2 tablespoons ground flaxseed

¼ cup water

2 tablespoons apple cider vinegar

1 teaspoon vanilla extract

¼ teaspoon sea salt

2 tablespoons maple syrup or coconut or date sugar

1 tablespoon plus 1 teaspoon baking powder

2 teaspoons baking soda

2½ cups Almond Milk (page 269)

3 cups white whole wheat flour

Zest of 1 lemon (optional)

½ cup or more fresh or frozen blueberries, preferably wild

Coconut oil, for greasing the griddle/ skillet

If you or someone in your family is allergic to eggs and dairy, you know how difficult it is to find good egg- and dairy-free foods that don't include cheap starches and refined sugars. The challenge of dealing with food allergies is even worse for parents when they cannot feed their kiddos some of the same basic foods that their friends eat. Well, when it comes to pancakes, this recipe is a game changer. These pancakes are so thick and fluffy, no one will ever guess that they don't contain eggs or dairy! Enjoy with your favorite pancake toppings.

In a large mixing bowl, combine the banana, flaxseed, and water, give the mixture a good stir, and let sit for 2 to 3 minutes.

Meanwhile, preheat a griddle or large skillet over medium heat.

Add the vinegar, vanilla, salt, and maple syrup to the mixing bowl and mix well. Add the baking powder and baking soda and mix well. (The mixture will react and start to fluff up.) Add the almond milk, flour, and zest, if using, and mix to form a thick batter (avoid overmixing). Gently fold in the blueberries.

Grease the griddle or skillet with coconut oil, scoop a few ¼-cup portions of the batter onto the hot griddle (as many as your griddle can take without overcrowding), and cook until the bottoms of the pancakes are golden, 2 to 3 minutes. Flip and cook the other side 1 to 2 minutes more.

Remove from the heat and repeat the process with the remaining batter. Serve.

NOTE: The pancakes freeze well. Before placing them in the freezer, separate them with parchment paper, then wrap in heavy-duty wax paper or aluminum foil. That makes it super easy to take out and reheat individual pancakes.

Savory Sheet Pan "Pancakes"

4 Yukon gold potatoes, peeled
2 carrots, peeled
2 scallions, thinly sliced
1 leek, well washed and thinly sliced
½ red bell pepper, seeded and diced
1 packed cup baby spinach, roughly chopped
¼ cup olive oil
4 large eggs
¼ cup Almond Milk (page 269)
1 teaspoon baking powder
2 teaspoons sea salt
1 teaspoon freshly ground black pepper
¼ cup whole wheat pastry flour
½ cup shredded cheddar cheese
½ teaspoon black cumin seeds or sesame seeds

This is one of my all-time favorite savory breakfast items. I created this recipe for a client's child—a picky eater who wouldn't touch any vegetables. I took some popular kid foods—potatoes, eggs, cheese, and milk—mixed them with some colorful veggies, then baked the mixture on a sheet pan. Cut into palm-sized rectangles, the resulting savory "pancakes" were a hit. They taste as good as they look and are filled with gut-friendly nutrients, including fiber and prebiotics. I like to use a box grater, but if you prefer a food processor or mandoline, that's fine. Make sure not to overblend with the food processor.

Preheat the oven to 350°F and line a large rimmed baking sheet with parchment paper.

Using the large holes of a box grater, grate the potatoes into a large mixing bowl. Do the same with the carrots in the same bowl. Add the scallions, leek, bell pepper, and spinach.

In a small bowl, whisk together the olive oil and eggs until well combined. Whisk in the almond milk, followed by the baking powder, salt, and pepper. Whisk in the flour until the mixture is lump-free, then pour it over the vegetables and gently mix until well-combined.

Transfer the mixture to the prepared baking sheet, spreading and flattening it evenly with a spatula. Bake for 25 minutes, sprinkle with the cheese and black cumin seeds or sesame seeds, and bake 20 minutes more or until lightly golden. Let cool slightly before slicing into palm-sized square "pancakes."

NOTE: The pancakes freeze well. Before placing them in the freezer, separate them with parchment paper, then wrap in heavy-duty wax paper or aluminum foil. That makes it super easy to take out and reheat individual pancakes.

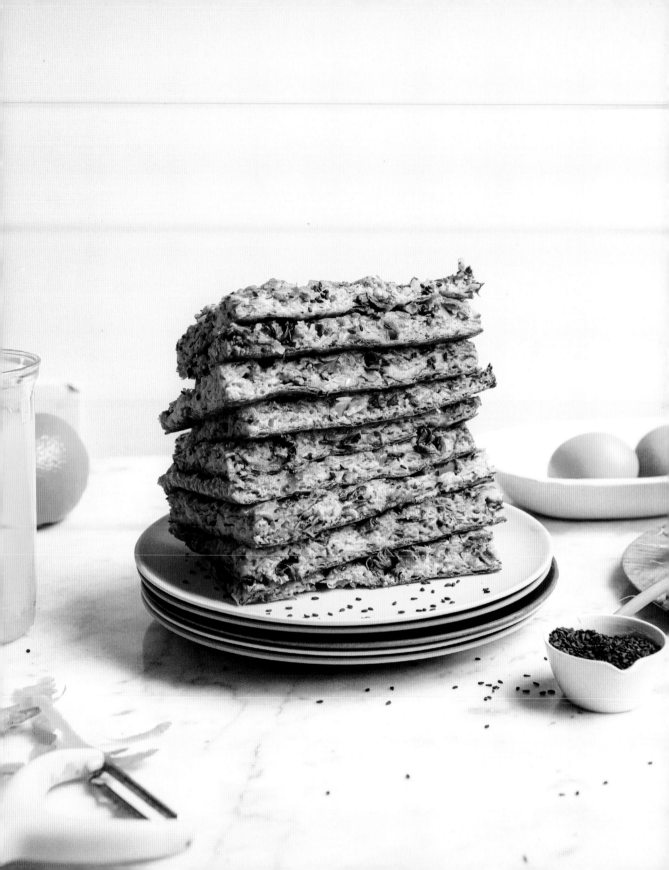

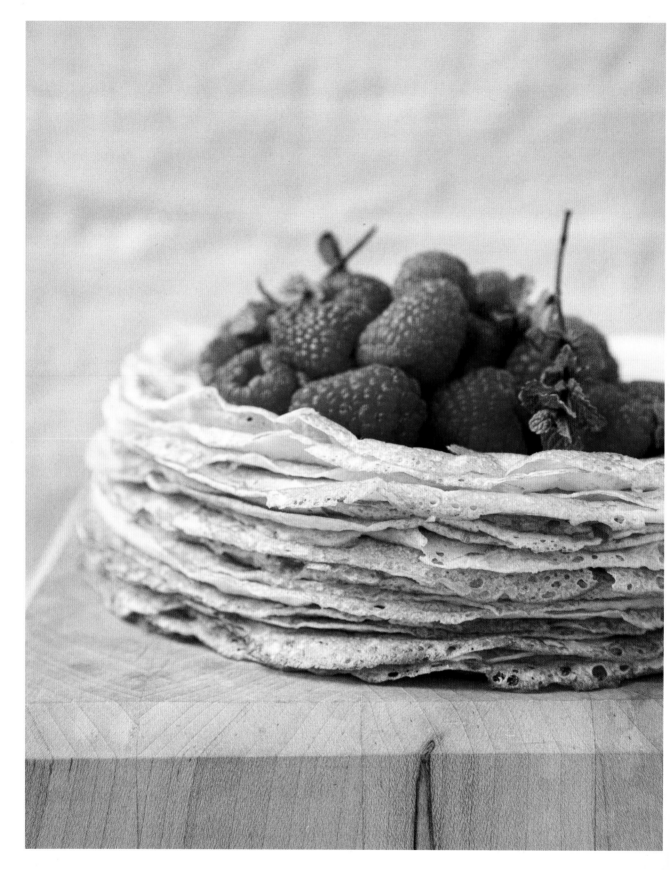

3 large eggs
2 cups Almond Milk
(page 269), Cashew
Milk (page 273),
Coconut Milk
(page 270), or Oat
Milk (page 274)
1 cup whole wheat
pastry flour
½ teaspoon freshly
grated nutmeg
¼ teaspoon sea salt
Melted coconut oil, for
greasing the skillet

Dreamy Whole Wheat Crepes

When I was growing up, crepes were a special treat, but after I moved into my own apartment, I began making them all the time. They are easy and quick once you get the hang of it, and everyone loves them. This crepe recipe, which uses 100 percent whole wheat pastry flour and coconut oil, is the result of much experimentation. Not only is it more nutritious than most versions, but the taste is also unbelievable. You can also make it gluten-free by substituting buckwheat flour.

Place all the ingredients except the coconut oil into a blender and blend until smooth. Let the batter rest for about 2 minutes.

Meanwhile, heat a 10-inch skillet (I use stainless steel; you are welcome to use what works for you) over medium heat.

Add coconut oil to coat the bottom of the skillet and pour any excess back into the container, making sure the oil is spread all over the pan. Pour ⅓ cup of the batter into the center of the pan and swirl gently to cover the entire bottom of the pan. Cook until tiny bubbles appear around the edge, 2 to 3 minutes. Flip and cook about 2 minutes more.

Transfer the crepe to a plate and repeat with the remaining batter, greasing the pan each time before use. Serve the crepes with fresh fruit and maybe a drizzle of maple syrup or your favorite toppings.

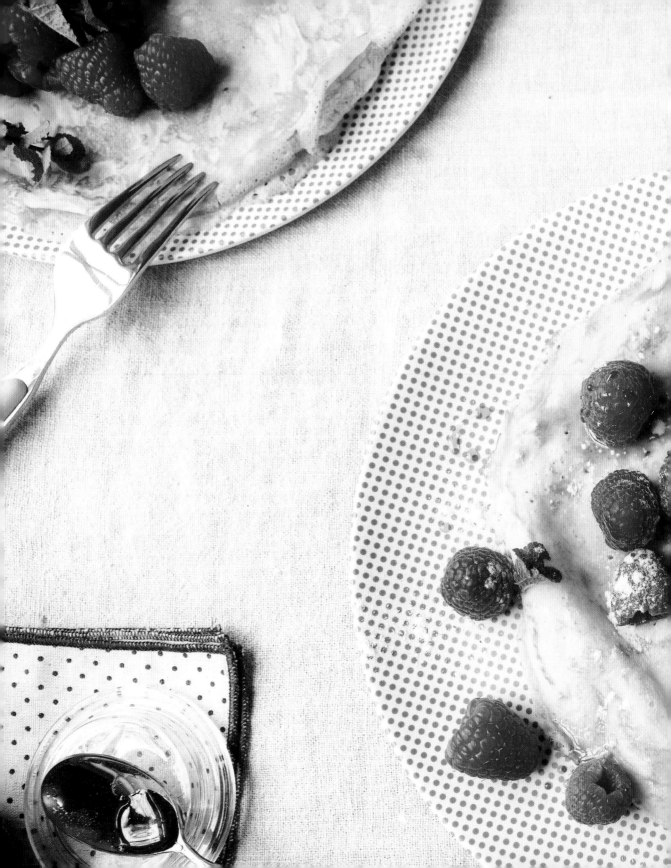

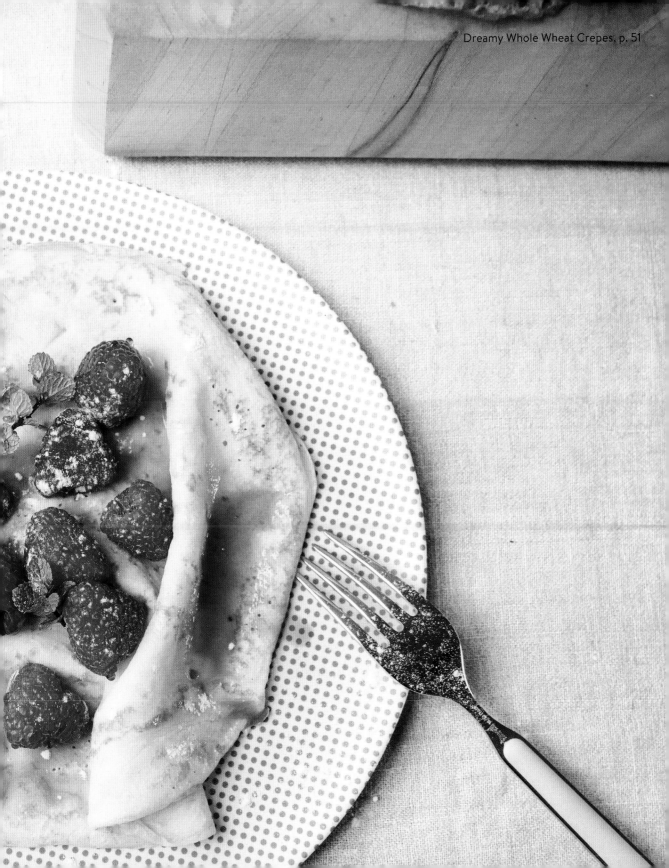

Dreamy Whole Wheat Crepes, p. 51

Sweet Potato Whole Wheat Waffles

SERVES 4 TO 6

3 tablespoons coconut oil, melted, plus more for greasing the waffle iron, if needed
2 cups whole wheat pastry flour
1 tablespoon plus 1 teaspoon baking powder
1 tablespoon sugar
1 teaspoon freshly grated nutmeg
½ teaspoon baking soda
1½ cups Almond Milk (page 269)
1 cup pureed sweet potato (see Notes)
1 teaspoon fresh thyme leaves
2 large eggs, whites and yolks separated

Although this recipe might sound a little odd, trust me—it's a real crowd-pleaser. Thanks to the whole wheat flour and sweet potato, these waffles are a nutritional powerhouse high in fiber and protein, too. The sweet potato lends sweetness and moisture, while the thyme rounds out the savory notes and adds a dose of immunity-boosting antioxidants.

Preheat a waffle iron. Depending on the type of iron you have, you may need to lightly oil it.

In a large bowl, combine the dry ingredients and whisk until well combined.

In a medium bowl, whisk together the milk, sweet potato, melted coconut oil, thyme, and egg yolks until well combined.

In a small bowl, beat the egg whites with a hand mixer at high speed until stiff peaks form when you lift the blades, about 2 minutes.

Pour the wet ingredients over the dry ingredients and whisk until well combined and nearly smooth, but do not overmix. Fold the beaten egg whites into the batter.

Cook the waffles according to the manufacturer's instructions. The amount of batter you use and the cooking time will depend on the your particular waffle iron. Enjoy these waffles with your favorite toppings.

NOTES: For the sweet potato puree: Bake a large sweet potato at 400°F until tender, about 1 hour. Allow it to cool, then peel and puree it in a food processor or blender, or simply mash it with a fork until smooth, adding a little water, as needed.

The waffles freeze well. Before placing them in the freezer, allow them to cool, unstacked, on a cooling rack. Wrap the waffles individually in parchment paper before placing them in a large resealable plastic bag. Heat in a toaster as you would regular frozen waffles.

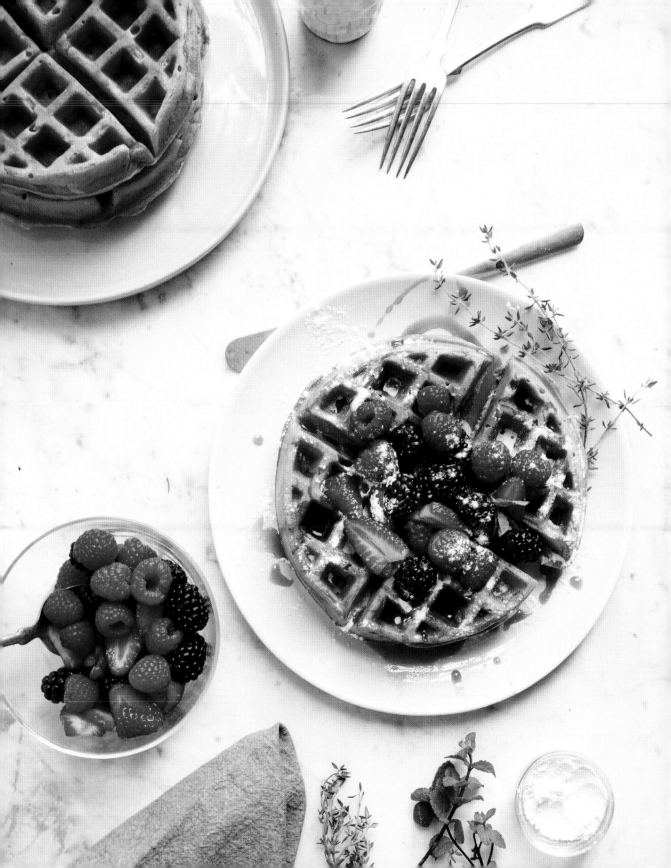

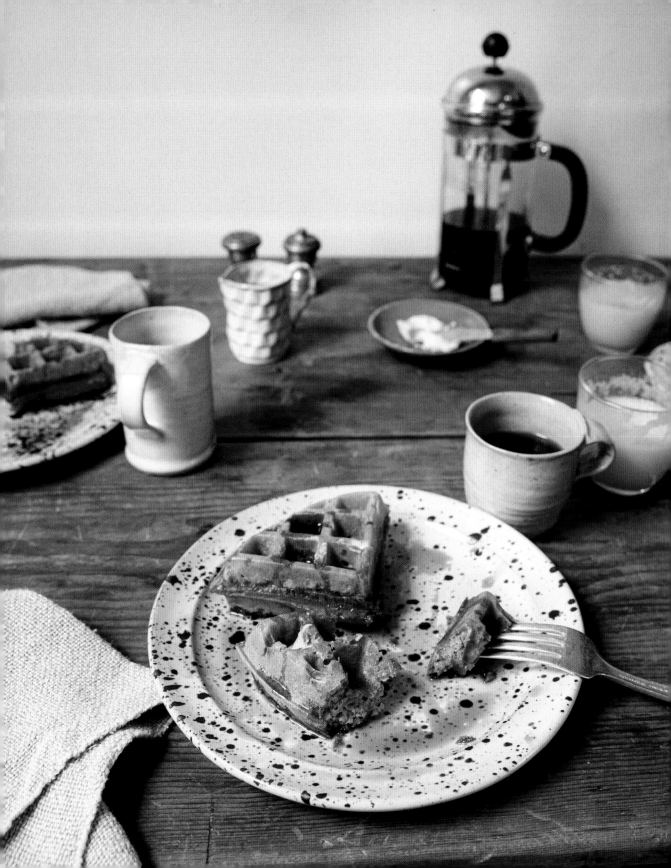

Quinoa Waffles

4½ cups quinoa flour
1 tablespoon plus
   1 teaspoon baking
   powder
2 tablespoons coconut
   or date sugar
1 teaspoon freshly
   grated nutmeg
1 teaspoon sea salt
4 large eggs
2½ cups Almond Milk
   (page 269)
1 cup olive oil
1 teaspoon vanilla
   extract
2 cups water
Coconut oil, for
   greasing the waffle
   iron, if needed

If you have ever tried to shop for healthy, delicious, and gluten-free waffles, you are going to have a deep appreciation for this recipe. These simple and delicious waffles are made without added starches, emulsifiers, or a load of sugar to fluff them up. They are made with light, nutritious quinoa flour, a superfood that contains all nine essential amino acids, making it a complete protein. You can get quinoa flour online if you can't find it at your local grocery store (though most stores carry it).

In a large mixing bowl, whisk together the dry ingredients.

In another large bowl, whisk together the wet ingredients.

Pour the wet ingredients over the dry ingredients and mix until well combined. Let the batter rest while you heat the waffle iron. Depending on the type of iron you have, you may need to lightly oil it.

When the waffle iron is ready, cook the waffles according to the manufacturer's instructions. The amount of batter you use and the cooking time will depend on your particular waffle iron.

Enjoy these waffles with your favorite toppings.

NOTE: The waffles freeze well. Before placing them in the freezer, allow them to cool, unstacked, on a cooling rack. Wrap the waffles individually in parchment paper before placing in a large resealable plastic bag. Heat in a toaster as you would regular frozen waffles.

Egg and Kale
Breakfast Quesadillas

GF

SERVES 2

4 large eggs
1 teaspoon onion powder
½ teaspoon sea salt
3 tablespoons olive oil, divided
½ onion, chopped
1 tomato, diced
1 clove garlic, minced
2 packed cups chopped baby kale
2 scallions, chopped
Ghee or olive oil, for greasing the skillet
4 corn tortillas or taco-sized flour tortillas
1 cup shredded cheese of your choice, such as Gruyère or cheddar

Not only is this dish absolutely delicious and easy to prepare, but it's also bursting with amazing nutrients for both the brain and the immune system. Kale is among the most nutrient-dense foods, and I always look for ways to add it to recipes.

In a medium bowl, whisk together the eggs, onion powder, and salt until light and foamy without any separation streaks of yolk or egg white.

In a medium skillet, heat 1 tablespoon of olive oil over medium heat until just starting to smoke, about 2 minutes. Add the eggs to the center of the pan and immediately reduce the heat to medium-low.

Wait for the edges to barely start to set, then using a spatula, gently push the eggs from one end of the pan to the other. Continue this process, pausing just enough between swipes to allow the uncooked egg to settle and cook, gently pushing the liquid to form the curds.

When the eggs are mostly cooked, with big pillowy folds, slowly fold the eggs in on themselves just a couple times, bringing them together. Move to a large plate and set aside.

In the same skillet, heat the remaining 2 tablespoons of olive oil over medium heat. Add the chopped onion and cook, stirring occasionally, until softened, about 3 minutes. Do not rush this step—it brings out the sweetness in the onion.

Add the tomato and garlic and continue cooking for about 2 minutes. Add the kale and scallions, reduce the heat to low, and cook, stirring occasionally, until the kale is softened, about 2 minutes. Remove from the heat and transfer to one side of the egg plate. Clean the skillet and return it to the stove.

In the cleaned skillet, melt a little ghee or olive oil over medium-low heat. Place a tortilla in the skillet and add one-quarter of the scrambled eggs, one-quarter of the cheese, and one-quarter of the kale mixture on one-half of the tortilla.

Fold the other side of the tortilla over the filling, press down on it with a spatula, and cook for 1 to 2 minutes. Flip and cook until the other side is crispy and golden, 1 to 2 minutes more.

Transfer to a cutting board and repeat the process with the remaining tortillas, scrambled eggs, cheese, and kale mixture. Cut the quesadillas in half and enjoy them warm.

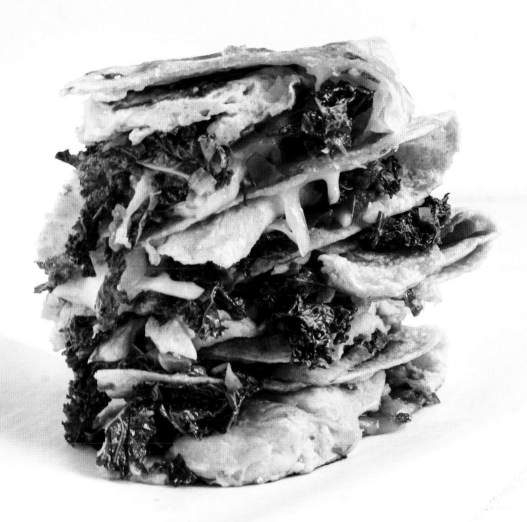

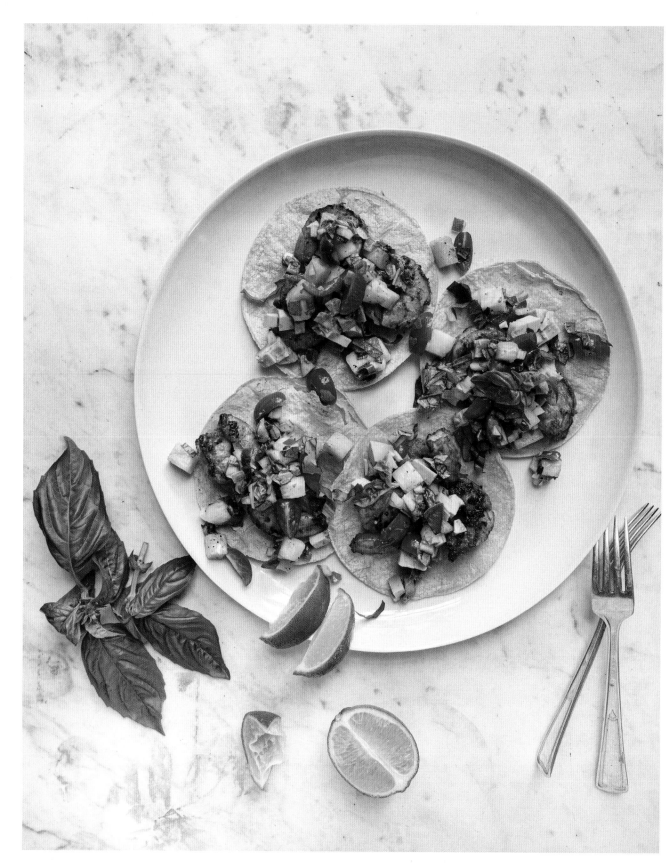

Shrimp Tostadas with Pineapple Salsa

This dish is packed with incredible flavors and is so fast and easy to make! As it's rich in brain- and immunity-boosting ingredients, such as wild-caught shrimp and avocado, I like to power-start my day with it, but the tostadas are great for lunch or dinner, too. Feel free to play with the ingredients in the salsa. Mango is a great substitute for the pineapple.

Preheat the oven to 400°F and line a large rimmed baking sheet with parchment paper.

For the salsa, in a medium bowl, mix together all the ingredients, then set aside.

For the tostadas, brush the tortillas on both sides with olive oil and place them on the prepared baking sheet. Bake until crispy, 8 to 10 minutes, flipping halfway through.

Meanwhile, in another medium bowl, toss the shrimp with the garlic powder, smoked paprika, cumin, salt, and pepper until evenly coated. Heat the oil in a large skillet over medium-high heat, add the shrimp, and sauté until pink and just cooked through, 2 to 3 minutes on each side.

Layer the tortillas with mashed avocado, shrimp, and pineapple salsa to serve.

PINEAPPLE SALSA

½ cup chopped pineapple
½ cup chopped cherry tomatoes
½ cup chopped red onion
⅓ cup fresh basil, chopped
Juice of 1 lime
½ teaspoon garlic powder
½ teaspoon sea salt, or to taste
¼ teaspoon freshly ground black pepper

SHRIMP TOSTADAS

4 corn tortillas
1 tablespoon olive oil, plus more for brushing tortillas
9 or 10 large shrimp, peeled and deveined
½ teaspoon garlic powder
½ teaspoon smoked paprika
¼ teaspoon ground cumin
½ teaspoon sea salt
¼ teaspoon freshly ground black pepper
1 ripe avocado, halved, pitted, peeled, and mashed

Sweet Plantains and Eggs with Spinach and Mushrooms

This dish—one of my favorites as a child—elevates the basic egg breakfast. It pairs eggs with roasted sweet plantains and sautéed spinach and mushrooms. It's filling, but not heavy, and super healthy: rich in iron, fiber, resistant starch, vitamins, antioxidants, and much more. Scale up the recipe when family and friends are visiting; they will be glad you did!

For the plantains, preheat the oven or an air fryer to 350°F.

In a large bowl, toss the plantains with the oil and salt, transfer to a sheet pan in a single layer or to the air fryer basket, and cook until brown, tossing halfway through, about 20 minutes total in the oven or 13 minutes in the air fryer.

Meanwhile, prepare the rest of the recipe. For the mushrooms, heat the oil in a large skillet over medium heat. Add the mushrooms and cook without moving for 2 minutes or until they start to glisten. Toss and continue cooking until golden brown, about 3 minutes more.

Add the butter, garlic, thyme, salt, and pepper to taste and cook, stirring occasionally, until the garlic is fragrant and the butter absorbs into the mushrooms, about 2 minutes. Transfer to a plate, reserving the skillet to cook the eggs.

For the eggs, pour the olive oil into the skillet and heat over medium low heat. Crack one egg at a time into the skillet, cover the skillet with a lid, and cook until the whites are set, 2 to 3 minutes. (If you prefer your eggs more well done, cook them longer. You can also cook the eggs separately if you don't want the whites to run together.) Season with salt, black pepper, and red pepper flakes, if using, to taste and transfer to one side of the mushroom plate.

Meanwhile, for the spinach, in the same skillet, heat the oil over medium-high heat. Add the garlic and cook, stirring, for 1 minute. Add the spinach, salt, and pepper and toss until the spinach is mostly wilted, 1 to 2 minutes. Serve with the plantains, mushrooms, and eggs.

PLANTAINS

2 ripe plantains, peeled and cut into bite-sized cubes
1 teaspoon olive oil
½ teaspoon sea salt

MUSHROOMS

1 tablespoon olive oil
8 ounces (about 2½ cups) portobello mushrooms, chopped or sliced
1 tablespoon butter
1 clove garlic, minced
2 teaspoons fresh thyme leaves
¼ teaspoon sea salt
Freshly ground black pepper

EGGS

1 tablespoon olive oil
4 large eggs
Sea salt
Freshly ground black pepper
½ teaspoon crushed red pepper flakes, or to taste (optional)

SPINACH

1 tablespoon olive oil
2 cloves garlic, minced
3 packed cups baby spinach
½ teaspoon sea salt
½ teaspoon freshly ground black pepper

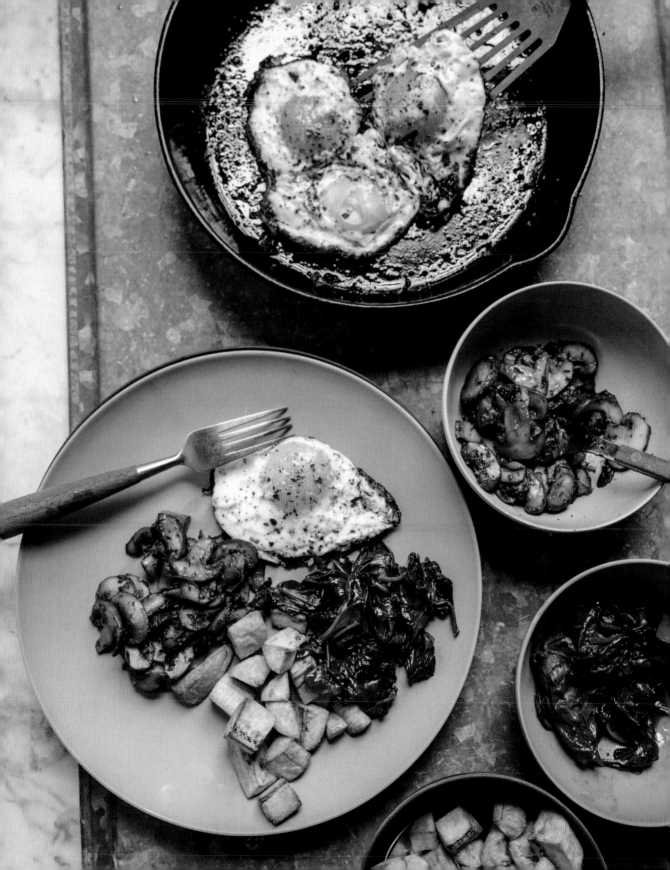

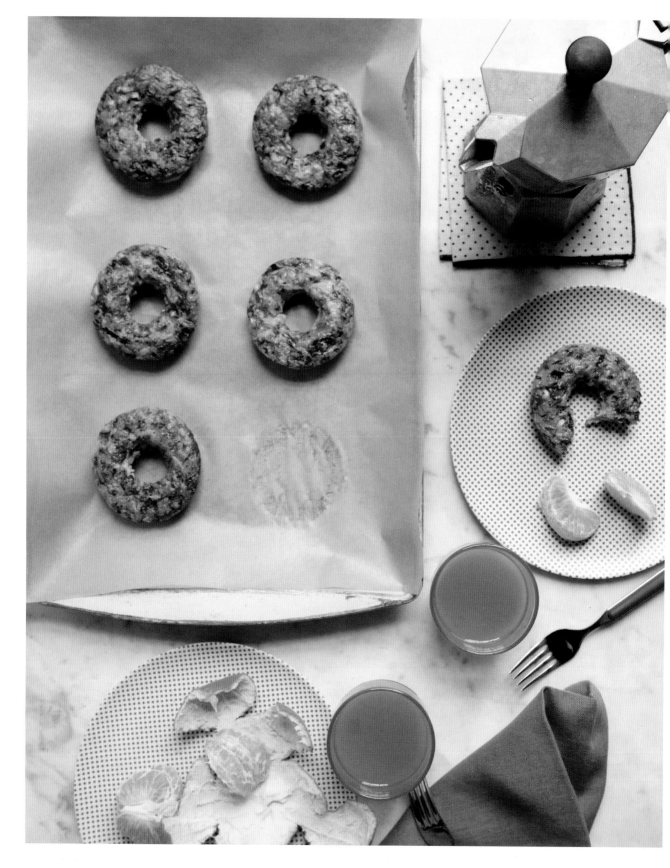

Tasty Omelette "Doughnuts"

Eggs are one of the very best sources of protein on earth, and one of the most easily digested. They are also high in omega-3 fatty acids, which are essential for brain development in infancy and childhood and brain health as we age. For those reasons and more, eggs are a good breakfast option to fuel us throughout the day. These colorful, doughnut-shaped individual omelettes are as tasty as they are pretty and will have both adults and children begging for more. (If you prefer to cook the egg mixture in a large skillet like a regular omelette, that's fine, too.)

2 tablespoons olive oil, plus more for greasing the doughnut pan
⅓ cup diced onions
⅓ cup diced red bell peppers
⅓ cup diced carrots
⅓ packed cup chopped spinach
2 tablespoons chopped fresh basil
⅓ cup shredded Gruyère or cheddar cheese
5 large eggs
3 scallions, thinly sliced
½ teaspoon sea salt, or to taste
¼ teaspoon freshly ground black pepper, or to taste

Preheat the oven to 350°F. Grease a 6-cavity doughnut pan lightly with oil and set aside.

In a large skillet, heat the oil over medium-high heat. Add the onions and cook, stirring occasionally, until translucent, about 3 minutes. Add bell peppers and carrots and cook, stirring occasionally, until tender, 3 to 4 minutes. Transfer to a mixing bowl and let cool.

Add the spinach, basil, cheese, eggs, scallions, salt, and pepper to the cooled mixture and mix well. Taste and adjust the salt and pepper as needed, then spoon the mixture into the prepared doughnut pan.

Bake until the eggs are just set, about 20 minutes, and let cool slightly before unmolding. Enjoy the "doughnuts" hot, warm, or at room temperature with a slice of bread, with a salad, or as is.

4 large hard-boiled
eggs
1 avocado, halved,
pitted, and peeled
1 tablespoon fresh
lemon juice
½ teaspoon sea salt,
or to taste
½ teaspoon freshly
ground black pepper
4 whole wheat
hamburger buns,
split and toasted
1 large tomato, thinly
sliced, about ¼ inch
thick
½ English cucumber,
thinly sliced
½ cup broccoli sprouts
or microgreens
All-Purpose Hot Sauce
(page 260) or your
favorite hot sauce
(optional)

Avocado and Egg Sandwiches

When I was a kid, I loved eating a chopped boiled egg seasoned with a little All-Purpose Hot Sauce (page 260) between slices of the fluffiest, thickest bread. When I think about that simple sandwich, I can still taste the delicious spiciness. This is an upgraded version that is a little more filling and nutritious. You can skip the hot sauce, if you like. For younger kids, I recommend mashing the mixture more finely and chopping the tomato. Also, for the kiddos, a milder delicious option for the hot sauce is to mix 1 teaspoon of sriracha with 3 tablespoons of plain yogurt, 1 teaspoon of fresh lemon juice, and a pinch of salt.

In a medium bowl, combine the eggs, avocado, lemon juice, salt, and pepper and mash with a fork until combined, leaving some chunks of eggs and avocado; do not overmix. Taste and adjust the seasoning as needed.

Divide the mixture evenly among the bottom buns. Top with tomato, cucumber, sprouts or microgreens, and hot sauce to taste, if using. Serve.

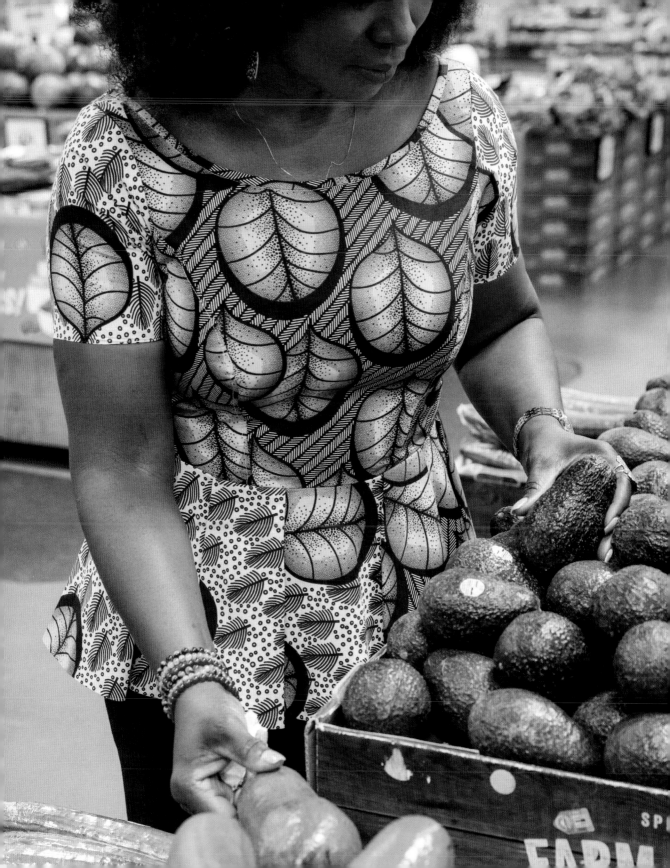

1 tablespoon butter
1 tablespoon coconut
  oil
1 tablespoon maple
  syrup
Zest and juice of
  1 orange
1 teaspoon vanilla
½ cup blueberries,
  preferably wild
½ cup raspberries
½ cup strawberries,
  hulled and quartered
½ cup blackberries
¼ teaspoon arrowroot
  powder (optional)
1 teaspoon water

Mixed–Berries Syrup

I am a firm believer that deprivation is not a sustainable practice. Children and adults alike love pancakes and waffles, so I needed to come up with a syrup that would keep everyone happy, since using ¼ cup maple syrup wasn't going to fly at our home. This syrup has been a gift that my family, clients, and social media family have all gladly embraced. I created this delicious "sauce" with a tablespoon of maple syrup, cold-pressed coconut oil, and butter to pull it all together; the berries turn a simple syrup into a tasty nutritional powerhouse. Use with Dreamy Whole Wheat Crepes (page 51), Egg- and Dairy-Free Blueberry Pancakes (page 47), or Sweet Potato Whole Wheat Waffles (page 54).

In a medium skillet, melt the butter and coconut oil over medium heat. Add the maple syrup and simmer for 1 minute, then add the orange zest and juice and vanilla and cook for 1 minute more.

Add all the berries and cook, stirring, until they begin to soften, 2 to 3 minutes; don't overcook the fruit. For a thicker mixture, in a small cup, stir together the arrowroot powder and water, then stir this slurry into the berries before removing from the heat. Top pancakes or waffles immediately. If saving, allow to cool, then transfer to an airtight container and refrigerate, covered, for up to 4 days.

NOTE: You can use fresh or frozen fruit. The cook time should be about the same.

2 cups frozen mixed berries
⅓ cup freshly squeezed orange juice
¼ cup maple syrup, or to taste
1 teaspoon fresh lemon juice
3 tablespoons water
1 teaspoon vanilla extract
1 teaspoon grated orange zest
¼ teaspoon freshly grated nutmeg

Wild-Berry Sauce

This is a delectable syrupy "sauce" I make and stash at home for super-special occasions. It is made with fiber-rich fruits bursting with incredible nutrients. I drizzle a teaspoon on a warm biscuit, plain yogurt, or bowl of fruit, or add it to nut butter sandwiches or warm homemade milk. It feels so silky and luxurious. Drizzle on Strawberry Ice Cream (page 110) or Tropical Vanilla Ice Cream (page 111).

In a small saucepan, bring all the ingredients to a boil over medium heat, then reduce the heat to low and simmer for about 10 minutes, crushing the berries with the back of a large spoon or a potato masher.

Remove from the heat, taste, and add more maple syrup, if you like. Pour the mixture through a fine-mesh strainer into a small bowl, pressing on the berries with a rubber spatula to release as much liquid as possible. (Save leftover pulp for smoothies or baked goods). Let cool, then transfer to an airtight container and store in the coldest section of the refrigerator for up to 3 weeks.

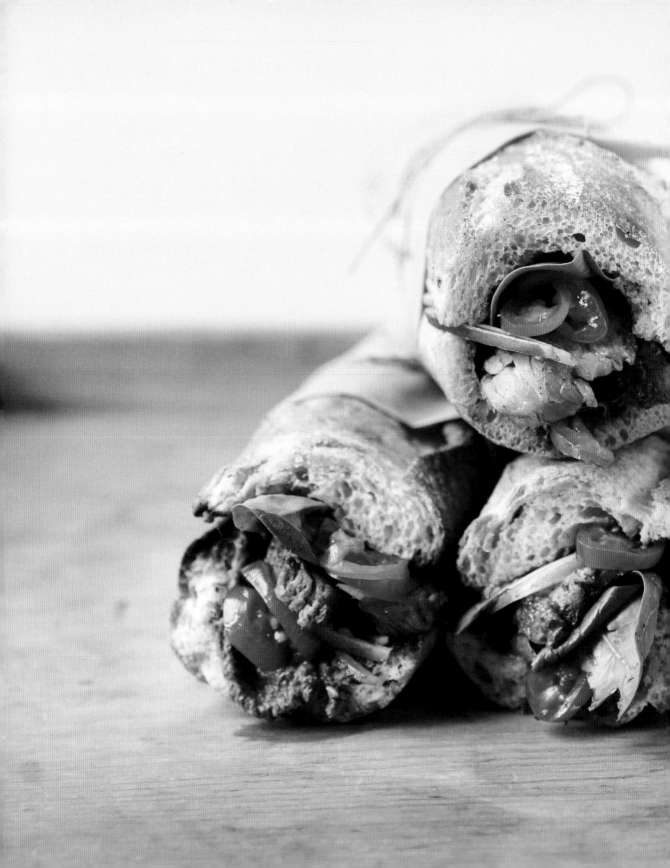

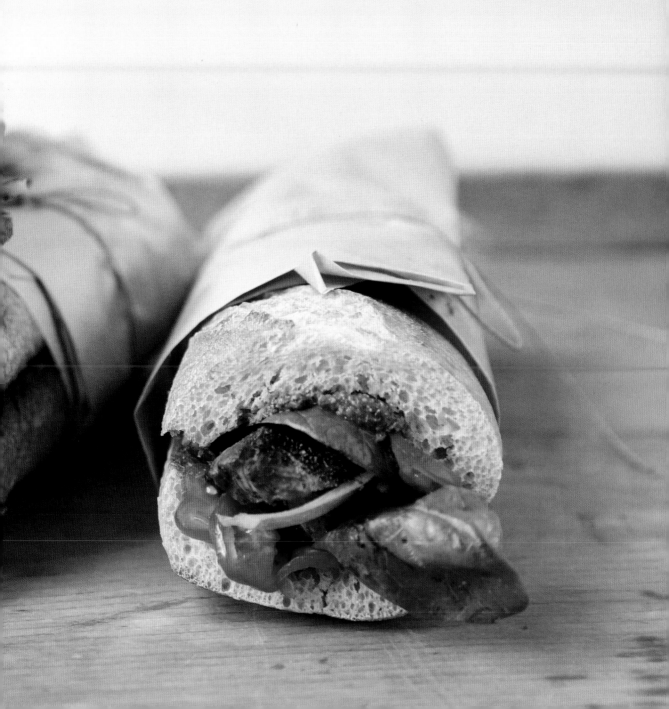

Portable Lunches

SANDWICHES ARE A LUNCHTIME staple for good reason. They are convenient and super easy to both make and eat in pretty much any setting. But, from a nutritional standpoint, sandwiches often lack nutrients. Eating processed meat and cheese on refined white bread with mayo isn't the best way to fuel up midday. In fact, a study published in the journal *Public Health* revealed that on days people ate a sandwich for lunch, they consumed more calories, fat, salt, and sugar than on days they didn't. It's also important to understand that what you eat for lunch also plays a big part in preventing that infamous mid-afternoon slump that no one wants, whether you are in an office, at home, or at school. But, here's some good news. I've pulled together some of my family's favorite lunches that are bursting with deliciousness, high in nutrients, and portable. Don't laugh, but I'm actually including three sandwiches. (Not all sandwiches are created equal!) These recipes might take a little more effort than you're accustomed to spending on lunch, but with a little extra planning, time, and resolve, I think you'll see the benefits are worth it.

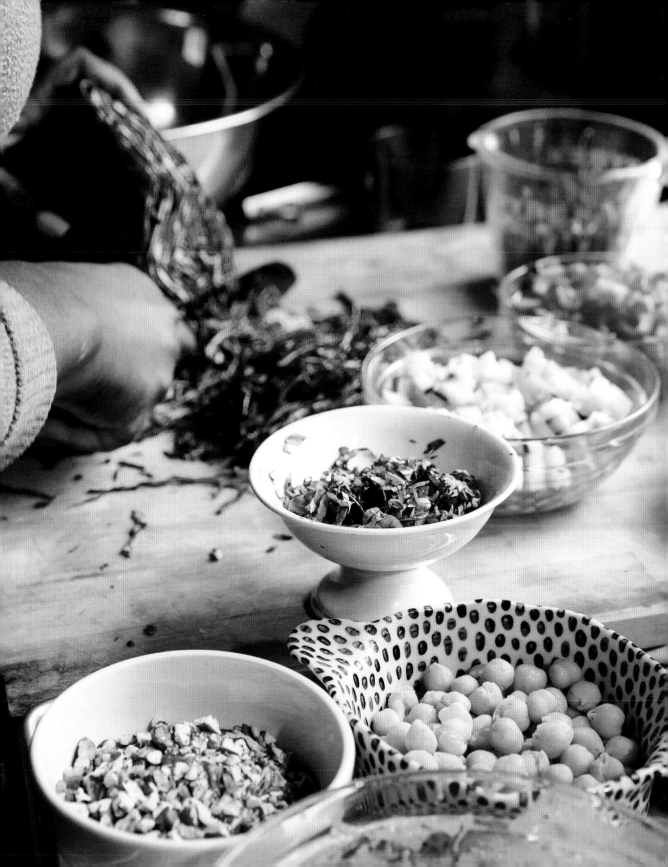

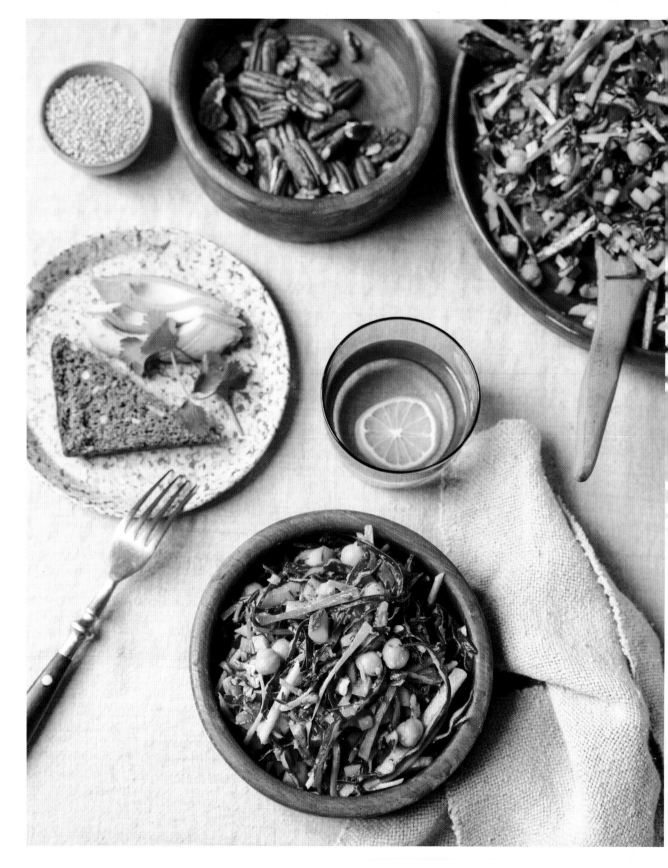

Protein-Rich Chopped Salad with Peanut Sauce

PEANUT SAUCE

- ¼ cup creamy peanut butter
- 3 tablespoons gluten-free rice vinegar
- 1 tablespoon maple syrup, or to taste
- 2 tablespoons fresh lime juice
- 2 tablespoons tamari or coconut aminos
- 1 tablespoon grated peeled fresh ginger
- 1 teaspoon toasted sesame oil
- ¼ teaspoon freshly ground black pepper, or to taste
- 2 cloves garlic, minced
- ¼ cup water
- ½ teaspoon crushed red pepper flakes (optional)
- Sea salt

SALAD

- 3 cups finely shredded cabbage
- 1 cup shredded carrots
- 1 cup cooked chickpeas, drained; if using canned, drained and rinsed
- 1 cup chopped cucumbers
- 1 cup shredded jicama
- 1 cup diced red and/or yellow bell pepper
- ½ cup chopped toasted pecans
- 2 tablespoons chopped fresh basil

When my friend April first tasted this salad, she burst out, "OMG, Agatha—this tastes amazing!" Every bite is an explosion of flavors and textures, thanks to the medley of vegetables, the toasted pecans (which also lend an extra dose of healthy fat), and creamy Asian-style peanut butter dressing. Even better, the salad is super healthy and filling. I promise it will become a new favorite in your home. I like to use my mandoline to cut the cabbage, carrots, and jicama and end up with the most beautiful salad.

For the peanut sauce, in a small bowl, whisk together all ingredients up to the water. Whisk in 1 tablespoon of water at a time until the consistency is just pourable, about ¼ cup total. Season to taste with red pepper flakes, if using, salt, and more black pepper. Set aside.

For the salad, in a large bowl, combine all the ingredients. Drizzle the dressing over the salad and toss to combine. Serve.

Tropical Shrimp Salad

3 tablespoons fresh
   lemon or lime juice
3 tablespoons olive oil
2 tablespoons gluten-
   free fish sauce
½ cup chopped fresh
   cilantro
1 pound precooked
   large shrimp, cut into
   thirds
1 medium jicama,
   finely julienned
1 ripe but firm mango,
   peeled, pitted, and
   cut into ½-inch
   chunks
1 small red bell
   pepper, thinly sliced
½ red onion, very thinly
   sliced
1 large avocado,
   peeled, pitted, and
   cut into ½-inch
   chunks
½ teaspoon crushed
   red pepper flakes, or
   to taste (optional)

This flavor-packed dish features nutrient-dense avocado, mango, and jicama, another unsung hero that contains many important vitamins and minerals, including vitamin C, folate, potassium, and magnesium. Combined with the omega-3 and selenium from the shrimp, this dish is a tasty winner when it comes to supporting immune-system health. It's great on its own, added to a poke bowl, with good toasted bread, or nestled in a lettuce wrap or taco shell. You can't go wrong with this one.

In a small bowl, whisk together the lemon juice, olive oil, fish sauce, and cilantro.

In a large bowl, combine the shrimp, jicama, mango, bell pepper, and onion. Drizzle the dressing over the mixture and toss to coat. Add the avocado and gently toss to incorporate. (If you're making this salad ahead of time, keep the avocado separate and toss it in just before serving.) Add the red pepper flakes, if using, and serve.

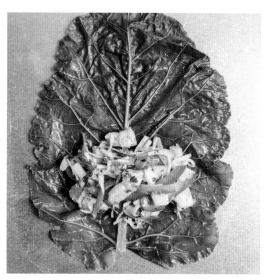
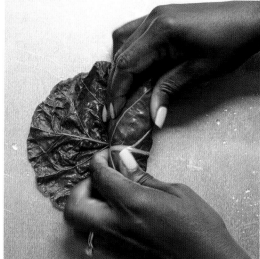

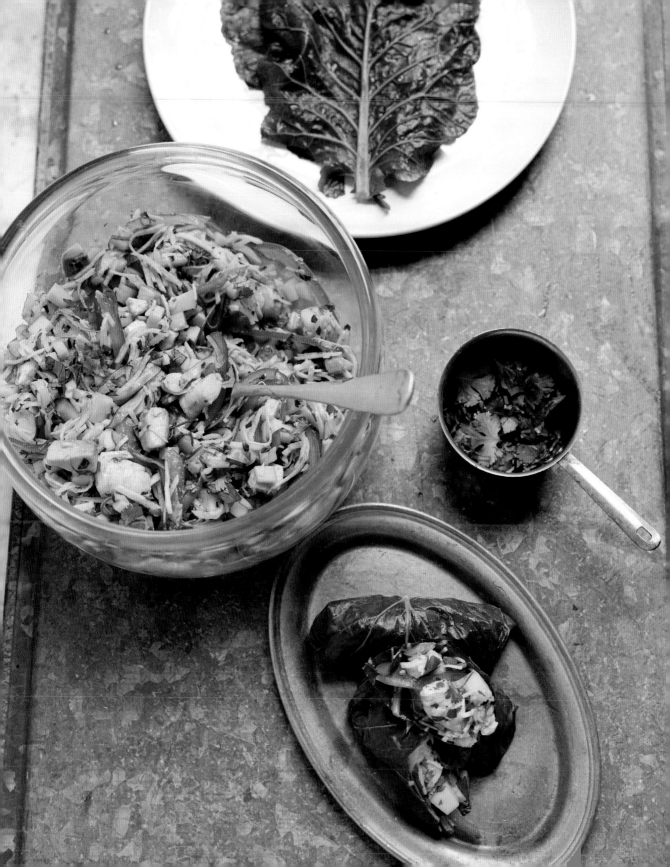

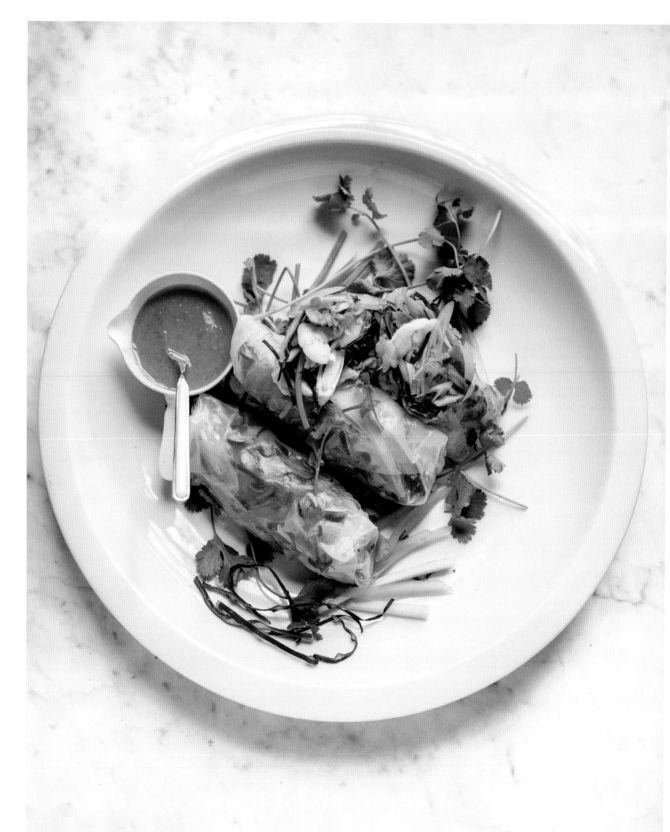

Shrimp Summer Rolls with Peanut Sauce

GF, DF

SERVES 4

SUMMER ROLLS

- 3 romaine lettuce leaves, quartered
- 2 cups microgreens, or 1 cup of your favorite sprouts
- 2 medium carrots, thinly sliced or julienned
- 1 cucumber, thinly sliced or julienned
- 1 yellow bell pepper, seeded and thinly sliced
- 1 cup finely shredded purple cabbage
- 24 (about 14 ounces) cooked large shrimp, peeled, deveined, and halved lengthwise
- 1/4 cup thinly sliced scallions
- 1/4 cup roughly chopped fresh cilantro
- 1/4 cup roughly chopped fresh mint
- 8 (8-inch) rice paper wrappers

Peanut Sauce (page 75)

With a little advance planning, this dish can be on the table in minutes. Simply prep all the components ahead of time and store tightly covered in the fridge. Then, all you need to do is assemble them. You can also let people make their own rolls. The blend of lettuce, purple cabbage, carrots, bell pepper, herbs, and shrimp wrapped in see-through rice paper sheets is really pretty and so clean and light—perfect for summer! And since you're using precooked shrimp, you don't even need to turn on the oven or stove! The rolls are wonderful for gut healing with their high fiber and water content. The sauce always goes fast. (My sons like to dip and twist their rolls in it, so I always make a double batch.)

Arrange all the ingredients up to the rice paper wrappers on a large platter.

In a large shallow dish, add about 1 inch of hot water. Place a rice paper wrapper in the water and let it soak until soft, but not super floppy, about 30 seconds. Carefully lay it flat on a clean flat surface, such as a cutting board or large plate.

Lay 1 piece of lettuce in the center of the paper, top with about one-eighth of the microgreens or sprouts, carrots, cucumber, bell pepper, cabbage, shrimp, scallions, cilantro, and mint. Fold the lower edge up over the filling, fold in the sides of the paper over the filling, and roll upward. Gently press the seam to seal. Repeat with the remaining ingredients and wrappers. Serve the summer rolls with the peanut sauce. If you aren't eating the summer rolls right away, cover with a damp paper towel, seal in an airtight container, and refrigerate for up to 2 days.

Shrimp Skewers with Kale Couscous

I am a little partial to this dish because couscous is one of the first foods from another culture I fell in love with at a very young age. It is still one of my favorites, although because we eat it so much, I cook 100 percent whole wheat couscous for that extra fiber. I toss the cooked couscous with kale, tomatoes, raisins, and lemon juice and top it with marinated shrimp skewers. It's a meal in itself, and a very easy and elegant one at that!

Preheat a grill to medium. You'll need 4 long or 8 short skewers, soaked in water for at least 30 minutes if using bamboo or wood. You can also cook the skewers in a skillet or grill pan on the stovetop with a little olive oil over medium heat, or broil them.

For the shrimp skewers, in a medium bowl, stir together the oil, lemon juice, parsley, garlic, salt, black pepper, and red pepper flakes, if using. Adjust the seasoning to taste. Add the shrimp and toss to coat.

Thread the shrimp onto the skewers and set aside any remaining marinade to brush on during grilling.

For the couscous, in a medium saucepan, bring the broth, oil, and ½ teaspoon of the salt to a boil over high heat. Add the couscous and raisins and stir, then cover, remove from the heat, and set aside for 5 minutes.

While the couscous rests, in a large bowl, combine the kale, tomatoes, scallions, lemon juice, remaining ¼ teaspoon of salt, and pepper to taste. Scrape and fluff up the couscous with a fork, add it to the bowl, and toss together.

Grill the shrimp until just cooked through, turning once halfway through and brush with the remaining marinade, about 5 minutes total. To serve, place the skewers on a bed of couscous or remove the shrimp from the skewers for an on-the-go lunch.

SHRIMP SKEWERS

- 3 tablespoons olive oil
- 1 tablespoon fresh lemon juice
- 2 tablespoons chopped fresh flat-leaf parsley
- 4 cloves garlic, minced
- ½ teaspoon sea salt, or to taste
- ¼ teaspoon freshly ground black pepper, or to taste
- ½ teaspoon crushed red pepper flakes (optional)
- 1 pound (20 to 25) jumbo shrimp, peeled and deveined

COUSCOUS

- 2 cups low-sodium chicken or vegetable broth
- 1 tablespoon olive oil
- ¾ teaspoon sea salt, or to taste, divided
- 1⅓ cups couscous
- ⅓ cup golden raisins
- 2½ cups stemmed and roughly chopped curly kale
- ½ pound (about 15) cherry tomatoes, chopped
- 2 scallions, thinly sliced
- 2 tablespoons fresh lemon juice
- ¼ teaspoon freshly ground black pepper, or to taste

Hummus Wraps

Way back in 1991, when I was in college, a classmate invited a few of us to come over to his family's house for a potluck dinner to celebrate International Students' Day. His aunty visiting from Egypt made hummus from scratch, which I had never had, and I was immediately hooked. Since then, I always tell friends that my introduction to that hummus was both a blessing and a curse. It was so good that if I want hummus, I have to prepare it myself because the store-bought versions just can't compare. For these wraps, I like to pair my homemade hummus with purple cabbage, orange bell peppers, scallions, and parsley in spinach or whole wheat tortillas. These wraps are so tasty, quick, and easy, especially if you decide to substitute with commercial hummus. (I'll never tell!)

For the hummus, combine the chickpeas, lemon juice, oil, tahini, cumin, garlic, salt, and pepper in a food processor, pulse until fairly smooth, scraping the side as needed. Taste and adjust the flavor to taste with more salt or lemon juice if needed and set aside.

For the wraps, in a medium bowl, mix together the lemon juice, oil, and pepper. Add the cabbage, bell pepper, parsley, and scallion and toss to coat.

Spread about ⅓ cup of the hummus on each of the tortillas, and top with about one-quarter of the cabbage mixture. Roll to close, tucking in the sides, then cut in half. Store any leftover hummus in the refrigerator for up to a week to enjoy with raw vegetables, such as carrots, bell peppers, and cucumber slices, or with warm pita bread.

HUMMUS

2 cups cooked chickpeas, drained; if using canned, drained and rinsed
3 tablespoons fresh lemon juice
2 tablespoons olive oil
2 tablespoons tahini
½ teaspoon ground cumin
2 cloves garlic, minced
½ teaspoon sea salt
½ teaspoon freshly ground black pepper

WRAPS

1 tablespoon fresh lemon juice
1 tablespoon olive oil
¼ teaspoon freshly ground black pepper
2 cups very thinly shredded purple cabbage
1 orange bell pepper, seeded and thinly sliced
¼ cup chopped fresh flat-leaf parsley
1 scallion, thinly sliced
4 (8- or 9-inch) spinach or whole wheat tortillas

Sardine and Avocado Sandwiches

2 (4½-ounce) cans
wild Pacific sardines
packed in olive oil,
drained
2 tablespoons salted
butter, at room
temperature
6 thick slices good-
quality sourdough or
whole wheat bread
1 small tomato, thinly
sliced
1 large firm but ripe
avocado, halved,
pitted, peeled, and
thinly sliced
6 fresh basil leaves,
thinly sliced
1 tablespoon fresh
lemon juice

Sardines are one of the most underrated superfoods, providing a good amount of iron, calcium (thanks to the edible bones!), and omega-3 fatty acids. They are also inexpensive, easily accessible, and a great pantry item, yet lots of people I've met in America have never tried them. I hope to change that with this dead-simple, really tasty, and very nutritious recipe. I pair the fish with avocado, which provides essential nutrients and phytochemicals and works synergistically with sardines to optimize health benefits.

In a small bowl, using a fork mash the sardines with butter until well combined. (The finished mixture reminds me of French pâté.) Do not remove the bones—they are loaded with nutrients and flavor.

Lightly toast the bread, then top 3 slices with the mashed sardine mixture, tomatoes, avocado, and basil. Drizzle with the lemon juice and top with the remaining slices of bread. Serve.

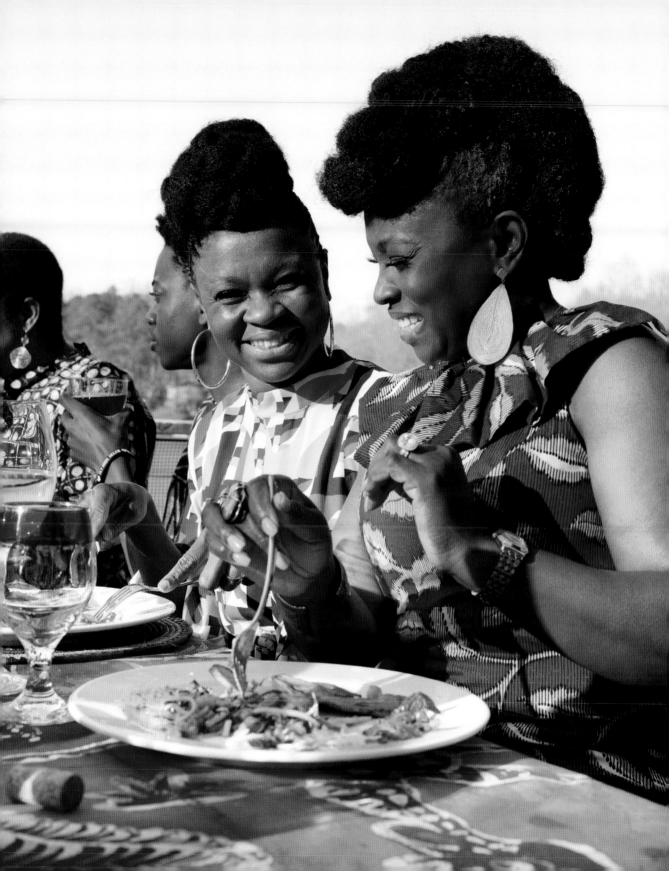

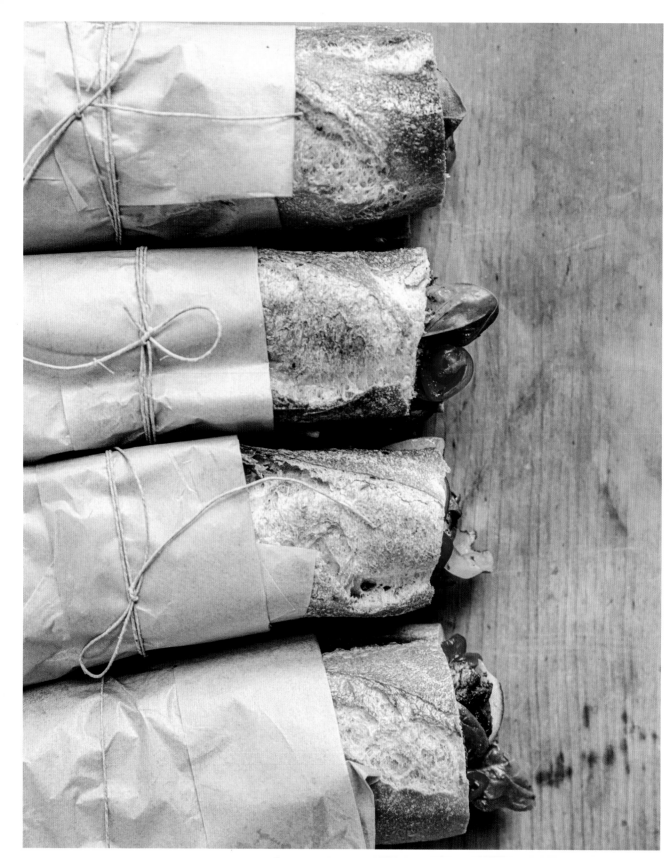

1 pound flank steak
3 tablespoons olive oil,
  divided
Sea salt
Freshly ground black
  pepper
2 packed cups baby
  spinach, divided
1 clove garlic, peeled
½ cup fresh basil
2 tablespoons freshly
  grated Parmesan
  cheese, preferably
  Parmigiano
  Reggiano
1 tablespoon fresh
  lemon juice
1 teaspoon drained
  capers
1 baguette, halved
  lengthwise and
  some of the soft
  insides removed
  from both halves
1 small red onion,
  thinly sliced

Skillet Steak Sandwiches

Now this is a sandwich with benefits: rich in protein, good fats, and antioxidants. The addition of fragrant basil-spinach pesto with the beef is unexpected and lovely. You can use kale instead of spinach if you prefer. You can also easily make the sandwich vegetarian by replacing the meat with your favorite mushrooms. (Oyster mushrooms are particularly good.)

Preheat the broiler to high.

Heat a cast-iron skillet or grill pan over medium-high heat. Rub the steak with 1 tablespoon of olive oil and sprinkle with salt and pepper to taste. Place the steak in the hot skillet and cook for about 4 minutes on each side for medium-rare. (Cook less if you want it rare and more if you want it well done). Transfer the meat to a cutting board and let rest for 6 minutes.

Meanwhile, make the spinach-basil pesto. In a food processor, combine ½ cup of the spinach, the garlic, basil, the remaining 2 tablespoons of oil, the cheese, lemon juice, and capers and process until the spinach is finely chopped. Set aside.

Place the baguette on a baking sheet cut-sides up and broil until lightly toasted, 1 to 2 minutes.

Thinly slice the steak against the grain. Layer the bottom half of the baguette with the remaining 1½ cups of spinach, sliced steak, and onion. Spread the pesto evenly on the top half of the baguette. This is where you can make this even more yours by adding a smidge of your family's favorite sandwich spread, though I will tell you my Turmeric Garlicky Mayo (page 259) will knock your socks off. Then place the bread on top of the sandwich. Cut into 4 pieces and enjoy.

Bunless Tofu Burgers

DF

SERVES 4

1 (14-ounce) package firm tofu, drained and pressed (see sidebar, below)
1 small carrot, finely diced
1 clove garlic, minced
¼ cup finely diced yellow bell peppers
¼ cup thinly sliced scallions
1 tablespoon chopped fresh flat-leaf parsley
1 teaspoon chopped fresh thyme leaves
2½ tablespoons whole wheat flour
1 teaspoon sea salt
1 to 2 tablespoons olive oil

Even fans of traditional beef burgers love these bunless tofu "burgers," chock-full of nutritious veggies and herbs, which lend texture, flavor, and color. Of course, you can serve them on buns, or in tortillas or pitas if you like. These can also be a quick snack meal for the kiddos to enjoy. Either way, pair them with the topping and condiments of your choice and a big green salad for a simple, delicious, beautiful, and healthful meal.

In a large bowl, mash the tofu with a wooden spoon or your hands. Add the carrot, garlic, bell peppers, scallions, parsley, thyme, flour, and salt and mix until well combined. Take about ⅓ cup of the mixture, gently shape it into a patty about 1 inch thick, and place it on a cutting board or large plate. Repeat with the remaining mixture.

In a large skillet, heat the oil over medium heat. Gently place the patties in the pan, in batches if necessary. (It's important not to crowd the skillet so you can easily flip the patties.) Cook, undisturbed, until hot and golden brown, flipping once halfway through, 6 to 8 minutes total and serve.

When you are sautéing or frying tofu or using it in dishes like these Bunless Tofu Burgers or Tofu and Mushrooms Stir-Fry (page 235), it's important to first remove as much excess water as possible. That way, it will hold up, brown, and crisp better, as well as spatter less when you add it to hot oil. It will have a denser, creamier texture, too. I generally use a tofu press, which is really convenient and easy, but here's a simple DIY method: Wrap a block of firm or extra-firm tofu (you don't press soft or silken tofu) in a clean dish towel or cheesecloth. Place a large plate upside down in a sheetpan, put the wrapped tofu on the plate, top it with a cutting board or casserole dish, and weigh it down with something heavy, such as large cans of tomatoes. (The sheet pan will collect the water as the tofu drains.) Let the tofu sit for 10 to 20 minutes, draining the water as needed. Unwrap and use as desired.

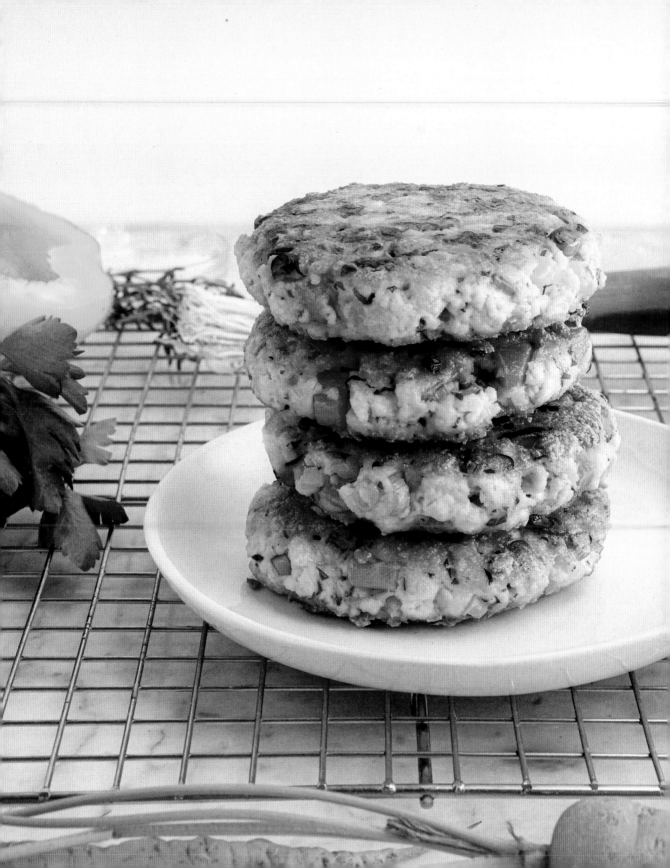

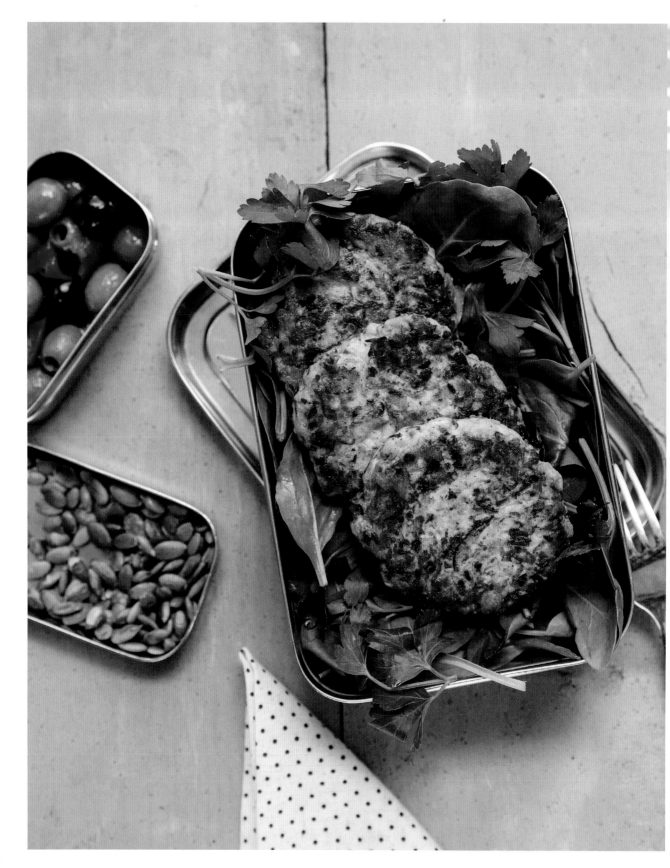

Salmon and Zucchini Patties

3 zucchini (1 to 1½ pounds), grated on the large holes of a box grater

1½ teaspoons sea salt, divided

1 pound salmon, finely chopped

5 scallions, thinly sliced

2 cloves garlic, minced

2 large eggs

⅓ cup finely chopped yellow onions

2 tablespoons chopped fresh flat-leaf parsley

¼ teaspoon freshly ground black pepper, or to taste

1 to 3 tablespoons olive oil

With the emergence of zoodles (zucchini noodles), zucchini quickly became the low-carb goddess alternative to pasta. But it's also a nutrient powerhouse, rich in vitamin A, fiber, and antioxidants. I like to combine grated zucchini with onions, scallions, garlic, eggs, and chopped raw salmon to make these moist, super-flavorful patties, which are delicious as is or as a sandwich/burger, especially topped with homemade mayonnaise, including my Turmeric Garlicky Mayo (page 259). Wild-caught salmon can be pricey, but I find frozen is cheaper, so I generally buy it that way. You can use a food processor to chop the salmon, but I prefer to do it by hand because I can better control the texture that way. If you use a food processor, be careful not to puree the fish.

Line a fine-mesh strainer with cheesecloth (if you have it), add the zucchini, toss with ½ teaspoon of sea salt, and set aside for about 15 minutes.

Meanwhile, in a large bowl, combine the salmon, scallions, garlic, eggs, onions, and parsley.

Squeeze the zucchini in the cheesecloth (or with your hands) to release as much liquid as you can. Add the zucchini to the bowl, then add the remaining 1 teaspoon of sea salt and the pepper and adjust to taste. Mix gently to fully incorporate all ingredients. Take about ⅓ cup of the mixture, gently shape it into a patty about 1 inch thick, and place it on a cutting board or large plate. Repeat with the remaining mixture.

In a large skillet, heat 1 to 3 tablespoons of oil over medium heat. Gently place the patties in the pan, in batches if necessary. (I cook 4 patties at a time in my large cast-iron skillet. It's important not to crowd the skillet so you can easily flip the patties.) Cook, undisturbed, until golden brown, 2 to 3 minutes. Flip the patties and cook, adding more oil if needed, until just cooked through and golden brown on the bottom, about 2 minutes more. Serve.

Chicken and Apple Kebabs

2 cloves garlic, minced
½ cup finely chopped fresh basil
⅓ cup gluten-free rice vinegar
2 tablespoons olive oil
1½ teaspoons raw honey (see Note)
4 teaspoons Dijon mustard
1 teaspoon fresh thyme leaves
1 teaspoon sea salt
¼ teaspoon freshly ground black pepper
4 boneless, skinless chicken thighs, cut into 1-inch pieces
1 zucchini, cut into ½-inch slices
1 firm apple, like Fuji or Gala, cut into ½-inch chunks
1 summer squash, cut into ½-inch slices
1 small red onion, cut into ½-inch slices

After working with families for so many years, I feel confident saying that even the pickiest eaters will enjoy, or at least try, this lunch, which is high in protein and antioxidants. For starters, kids (and adults!) generally love food on a stick. It's fun and interesting to look at and to eat. The combo of chicken and apple is popular, too. And after some experimentation, I added both green and yellow squash because while some kids have an aversion to green vegetables, they might eat yellow ones. It's always interesting to see what parts of the kebab are passed over. See what works best for your family and prepare them accordingly. I like to serve the kebabs with rice and salad.

Preheat a grill to medium. You'll need 4 long or 8 short skewers, soaked in water for at least 30 minutes if using bamboo or wood. You can also cook the kebabs in a skillet or grill pan on the stovetop with a little olive oil over medium heat, or broil them.

In a small bowl, combine the garlic, basil, vinegar, oil, honey, mustard, thyme, salt, and pepper, then whisk together with a fork and set aside.

Assemble the skewers in the following order: a piece of chicken, zucchini, apple, squash, then onion. If you can fit a few more ingredients on each skewer, that's fine. Brush the basil mixture on the skewers and grill the kebabs, turning occasionally, until the chicken is just cooked through, 12 to 14 minutes, and serve. For an on-the-go lunch, remove the ingredients from the skewers.

NOTE: Do not serve raw honey to babies twelve months or younger, as it may cause infant botulism. Use mustard flavored with maple syrup instead.

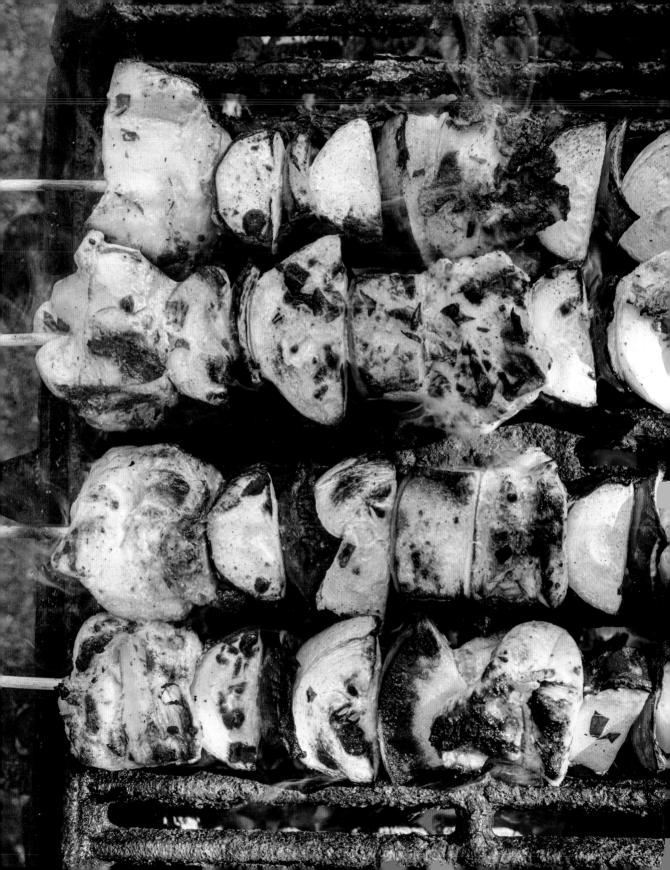

Chicken and Vegetable Hand Pies

These scrumptious, super-nutritious hand pies, made with whole wheat pastry flour, travel so well, they are our go-to for long flights. The chicken, green bean, carrot, and pea filling is great, but you can basically use whatever protein (beef, shrimp, tofu, etc.) and veggies you like. The flaky dough is easy to prepare, but if necessary, substitute with ready-made pie dough you find in the refrigerated or frozen section of your local grocery store. The dough and the pies freeze well, and any unused portion should be tightly wrapped and can be stored for up to 5 months.

For the dough, in a small bowl or cup, combine the water and ice cubes and allow the cubes to melt a little to make the water even colder (this helps create a tender, flaky result).

Sift the flour and salt into a food processor and pulse 3 to 5 times. Add the butter and pulse until the mixture resembles a coarse meal with some pea-sized pieces of butter.

With the food processor running, add 1 tablespoon of the water at a time through the chute until a dough forms (you may only need about 7 tablespoons of water, so watch the dough closely). Turn the dough out onto a lightly floured surface and knead for just about a minute. Form the dough into a ball, divide it into 4 balls, and wrap in plastic wrap. Place in the refrigerator for about 30 minutes.

Meanwhile, preheat the oven to 400°F. Line a baking sheet with parchment paper and set aside.

For the filling, in a large skillet, heat the oil over medium-high heat. Add the onion and cook, stirring occasionally, until tender, 2 to 3 minutes. Add the green beans, carrots, thyme, and garlic and cook, stirring occasionally, until the vegetables are tender, about 5 minutes more. Add the chicken and peas, then sprinkle in the flour and stir to coat the vegetables.

DOUGH

- ½ cup ice water plus 10 ice cubes
- 2 cups whole wheat pastry flour, plus more for rolling out the dough
- 1 teaspoon sea salt
- 6 tablespoons (¾ stick) cold butter, cut into ½-inch cubes

FILLING

- 2 tablespoons olive oil
- ½ red onion, diced
- ½ cup thinly sliced (about ¼ inch) green beans
- ½ cup finely diced (about ¼ inch) carrots
- 1 tablespoon chopped fresh thyme leaves
- 2 cloves garlic, minced
- 2 cups shredded cooked white meat from a rotisserie chicken or from Roasted Chicken (page 157)
- ½ cup fresh or frozen green peas
- 2 tablespoons whole wheat pastry flour
- 1½ cups low-sodium chicken broth
- 1 tablespoon chopped fresh flat-leaf parsley
- ¼ teaspoon freshly ground black pepper
- ½ teaspoon sea salt, or to taste
- 1 large egg, beaten with 1 tablespoon water

Stir in the chicken broth and bring to a boil. Cook, stirring occasionally, until thickened, about 3 minutes. Fold in the parsley, pepper, and ½ teaspoon salt. Adjust the seasoning to taste and set aside.

Remove the dough from the refrigerator and allow to rest at room temperature for 5 minutes.

Divide each of the 4 balls in half (for 8 large hand pies) or in quarters (for 16 small hand pies). On a lightly floured surface, roll each ball into a circle. (It doesn't have to be perfect.) Spoon about ⅓ cup (for a large pie) or 1 heaping tablespoon (for a small pie) of the filling into the center of each circle.

Fold the dough over the filling to form a half-moon. Crimp the edges with your fingers to seal, then lightly press down on the border with the tines of a fork. Cut two slits in the top of each pie with a sharp knife or simply use the fork. Place the pies on the prepared pan, brush the tops with beaten egg wash, and bake until the crust is lightly browned, 20 to 25 minutes.

Serve.

Silence the voices that tell you making homemade pie dough is hard or not worth it. Trust me—it is worth it and neither the baking equivalent of Mt. Everest nor time-consuming, especially if you use a food processor. Follow the process in my Chicken and Vegetable Hand Pies (page 92) and you'll have brag-worthy dough in a grand total of 10 minutes. You can also use the dough for quiche, pot pie, and cobbler.

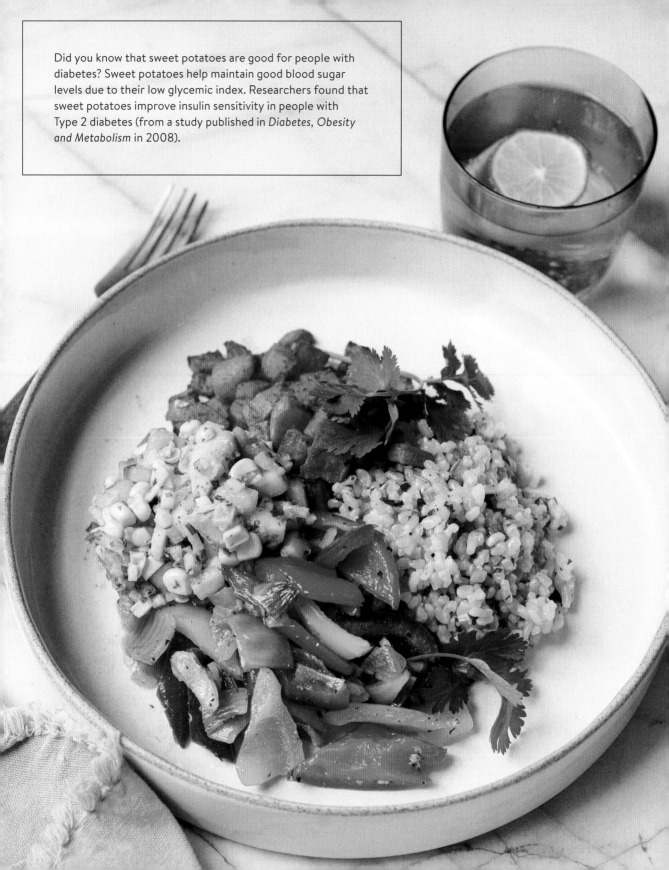

Did you know that sweet potatoes are good for people with diabetes? Sweet potatoes help maintain good blood sugar levels due to their low glycemic index. Researchers found that sweet potatoes improve insulin sensitivity in people with Type 2 diabetes (from a study published in *Diabetes, Obesity and Metabolism* in 2008).

Roasted-Vegetable Burrito Bowls with Pineapple Avocado Salsa

GF, DF

SERVES 4

I love making these burrito bowls—our home is filled with the most delightful smell when the vegetables are roasting. Sweet potatoes are a key ingredient here. Not only do they taste particularly good roasted, but they are also low in calories and are a healing food, rich in fiber, vitamins, potassium, proteins, and essential nutrients. The pineapple salsa makes the dish even more nutritious and is great with tortilla chips, on fish tacos, and the like. Instead of making a bowl, you can wrap the vegetables and rice in a warm tortilla and serve with the salsa on the side, if you prefer.

Preheat the oven to 390°F. Line a sheet pan with parchment paper.

For the vegetables, in a large bowl, toss together the sweet potatoes, 2 tablespoons of the oil, smoked paprika, coriander, cumin, and salt and pepper to taste. Spread the sweet potatoes out on one side of the prepared sheet pan, reserving the bowl.

In the same bowl, toss together the bell peppers, onion, garlic, oregano, and salt and pepper to taste. Spread the vegetables out on the empty part of the baking sheet, leaving a little space between the two sides. Bake until the vegetables are tender and caramelized, about 30 minutes, flipping midway for even cooking.

Meanwhile, for the salsa, in a medium bowl, gently toss together the avocado, cucumber, corn, jicama, pineapple, cilantro, and lemon juice.

When the vegetables are ready, place the rice at the bottom of each bowl and top with the roasted vegetables and pineapple avocado salsa. Serve.

VEGETABLES AND RICE

1 large sweet potato, peeled and diced into 1-inch chunks
¼ cup olive oil, divided
1 teaspoon smoked paprika
½ teaspoon ground coriander
½ teaspoon ground cumin
Sea salt
Freshly ground black pepper
1 green bell pepper, seeded and chopped
1 red bell pepper, seeded and chopped
1 yellow bell pepper, seeded and chopped
1 red onion, chopped
2 cloves garlic, minced
1 teaspoon dried oregano
1 cup steamed brown rice

SALSA

1 avocado, pitted, peeled, and cut into ½-inch cubes
½ cup diced cucumber (about ½ inch)
½ cup fresh sweet corn
½ cup diced jicama (about ½ inch)
½ cup diced pineapple (about ½ inch)
2 tablespoons chopped fresh cilantro
Juice of 1 lemon

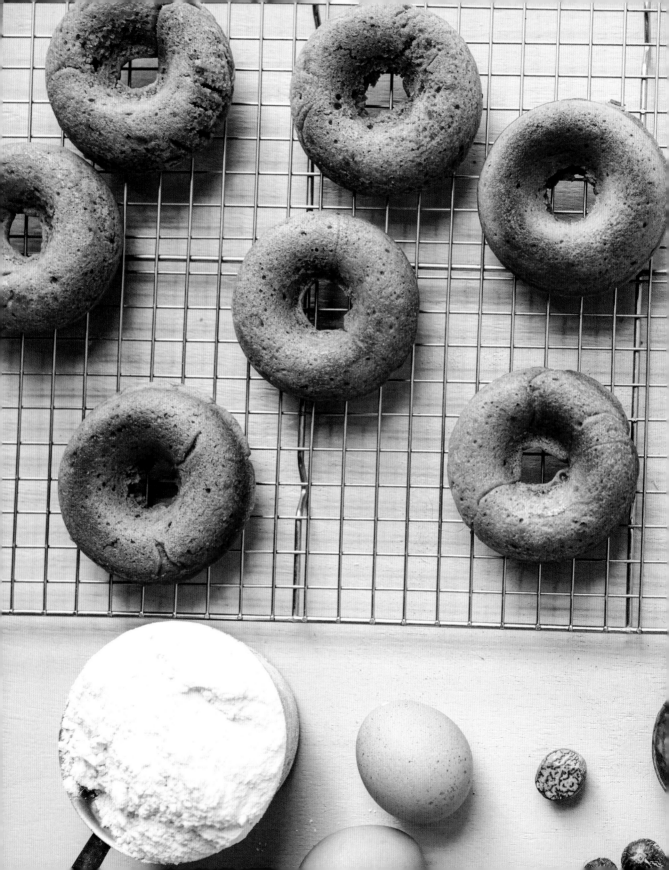

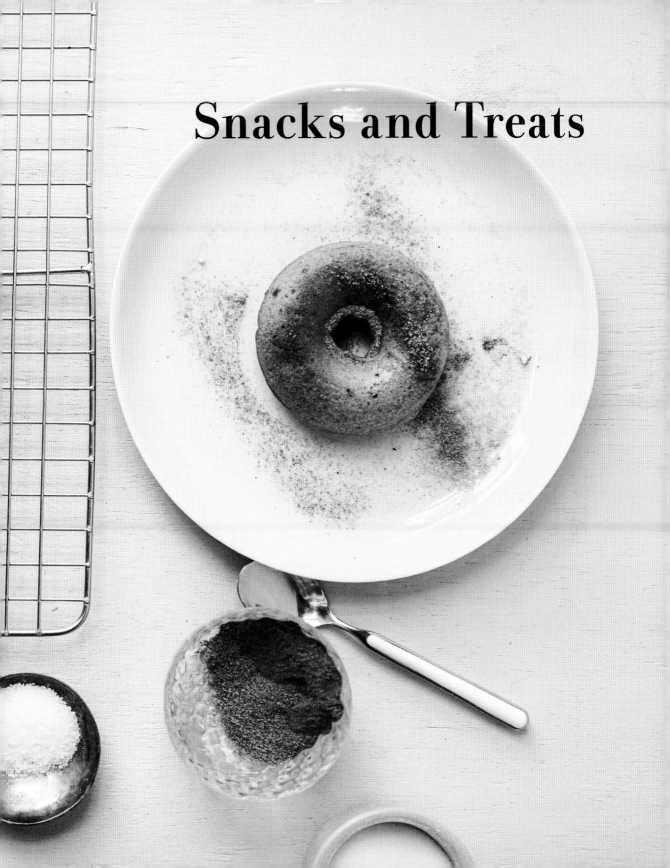

Snacks and Treats

THERE IS A HUGE DIFFERENCE between a snack and a treat. A snack is (or should be!) a healthy bite between meals, while a treat is a once-in-a-while celebratory food. Helping our families, especially the children, understand this distinction will serve them for life.

The truth is, children with their tiny tummies need snacks to fill in the gaps between meals. Giving them healthy, nutrition-packed snacks ensures that kids of all ages (especially toddlers during their picky-eating phase) get more of the vitamins, minerals, antioxidants, essential fats, protein, and fiber needed for developing brains and bodies. It's also a great opportunity to help train kids' palates to enjoy a wide variety of healthy flavors. And foods they might not eat at the table are sometimes given a chance in a different setting or while on the go.

A treat doesn't necessarily have real health benefits, but it satisfies a craving for sweet or salty foods, and it makes us happy, which is also very important. However, because treats generally have very little or no nutritional value, we don't allow them every day and do not stock them at home. We buy or make them for special celebrations.

The same goes for adults! I cannot tell you how many thousands of parents have told me that sharing that approach to snacks and treats has been life-changing—not just for their children, but for themselves as well.

Here are some of my family's favorite homemade snacks and treats. Every one of them is healthy (sometimes, all it takes are a few twists) and easy to make and has been called delicious by people other than me. That last adjective is really important—I strongly believe there's no point in packing nutrients into recipes if you are compromising on taste.

1 cantaloupe, the flesh cut into cubes, or balls with a melon baller

1 honeydew, the flesh cut into cubes, or balls with a melon baller

1 mango, the flesh cut into cubes, or balls with a melon baller

½ watermelon, the flesh cut into cubes, or balls with a melon baller

¼ pineapple, the flesh cut into bite-sized chunks

Juice of 2 oranges

Juice of 1 lemon

⅓ cup raw honey (see Note)

½ teaspoon vanilla extract

Fresh Fruit Salad, a.k.a. Vitamin C in a Bowl

This salad—a combo of seven types of fruit—always disappears minutes after I put it on the table. Not only is it a crowd-pleaser, it's also a power-packed dose of fiber, vitamins, and antioxidants. You don't just get a wider variety of nutrients by eating more types of fruits—those nutrients actually work together to produce even more powerful health benefits than any single fruit can alone. Think of it like compounding interest—but with fruit! If you're making melon balls, get the kiddos (if they are the appropriate age) in on the action. Their scoops may not be perfect, but they will have so much fun practicing and improving their motor skills. You, on the other hand, will have help without worrying about them handling a knife.

In a large bowl, combine the cantaloupe, honeydew, mango, watermelon, and pineapple and set aside while you make the sauce.

In a saucepan, bring the orange juice, lemon juice, honey, and vanilla to a boil over high heat, whisking until the honey is incorporated. Reduce the heat to low and simmer, stirring occasionally, until slightly thickened, about 6 minutes. Set aside until cool, about 10 minutes.

Pour the sauce over the fruit and gently toss to coat. Refrigerate, covered, for at least 4 hours. Serve.

NOTE: Do not serve raw honey to babies twelve months or younger, as it may cause infant botulism. Use maple syrup instead.

Strawberry Chia Pudding

10 large strawberries, hulled and sliced
1 cup milk of your choice
1 tablespoon raw honey, or to taste (see Note)
1 teaspoon vanilla extract
¼ cup chia seeds
Toppings of choice (berries, granola, sliced banana, nuts, hemp seeds, etc.)

This is a super-easy and popular make-ahead snack that is also great for breakfast. If you are not already a fan of chia seeds, here's the perfect starter recipe. There are so many amazing benefits to this seed (rich in protein, omega-3 fatty acids, fiber, minerals, and antioxidants), and you can just sprinkle them into smoothies, oatmeal, salads, soups, and pancake/muffin batters, to name a few uses, so a bag goes quickly in my house. I like to use strawberries in the pudding for health benefits (and a beautiful color), but you can use whatever fruit you prefer.

In the cup of a blender, blend the strawberries, milk, honey, and vanilla on high speed until smooth. Taste and add a little more honey, if needed. Pour into a glass jar or container with a lid.

Mix in the chia seeds, wait 5 minutes, and stir again. Refrigerate, covered, for at least 3 hours or overnight for best results.

Serve in small bowls with your favorite toppings.

NOTE: Do not serve raw honey to babies twelve months or younger, as it may cause infant botulism. Use maple syrup instead.

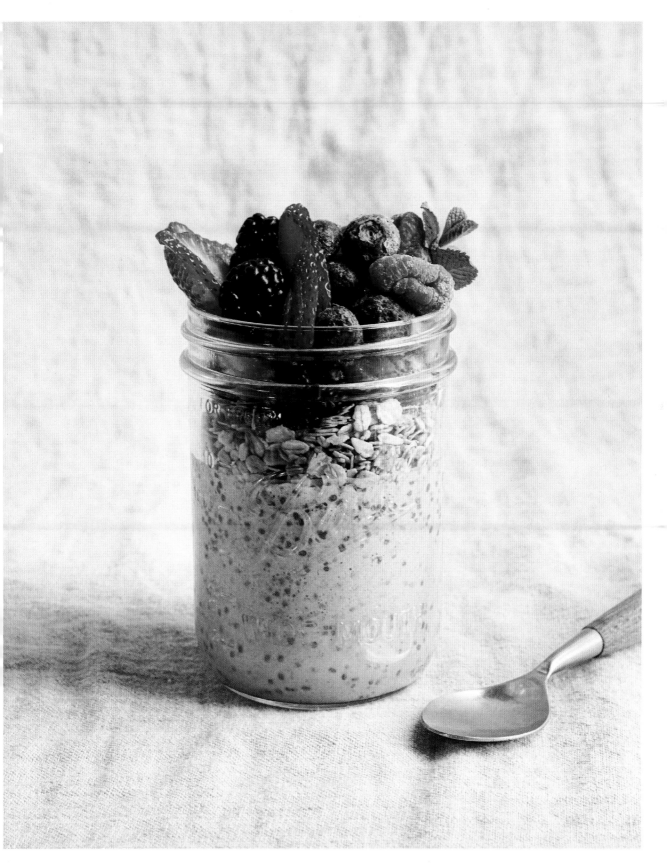

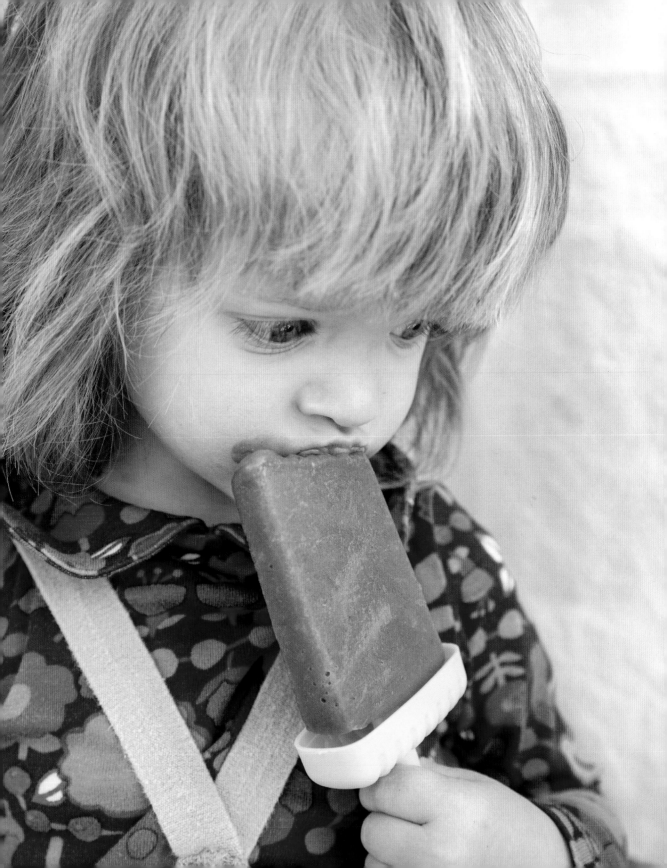

1 ripe banana, peeled
  and sliced
1 mango, peeled and
  diced
2 cups baby spinach
1 cup pineapple
  chunks
Juice of 1 orange
Juice of ½ lemon

Mango and Pineapple Popsicles

If you have a picky eater who won't touch anything green, these ice pops may very well change that. They taste so good and are super-hydrating. They are also packed with nutrients and anti-inflammatory properties. And unlike many commercial ice pops, they don't have any added sugars or artificial or synthetic ingredients.

In a blender, combine all the ingredients and blend on high speed until smooth. Pour into 6 ice-pop molds (see Note), being careful not to overfill. Insert the sticks/tops and freeze overnight before serving.

NOTE: I use an ice-pop mold with 6 compartments. You can use whatever size you like, but note that the fill and yield amount may be different. If you don't have an ice-pop mold, use 3- to 5-ounce paper cups. Fill the cups with the mixture, then cover each with foil, cut a slit in the center, and insert a wooden ice-pop stick. Freeze on a tray.

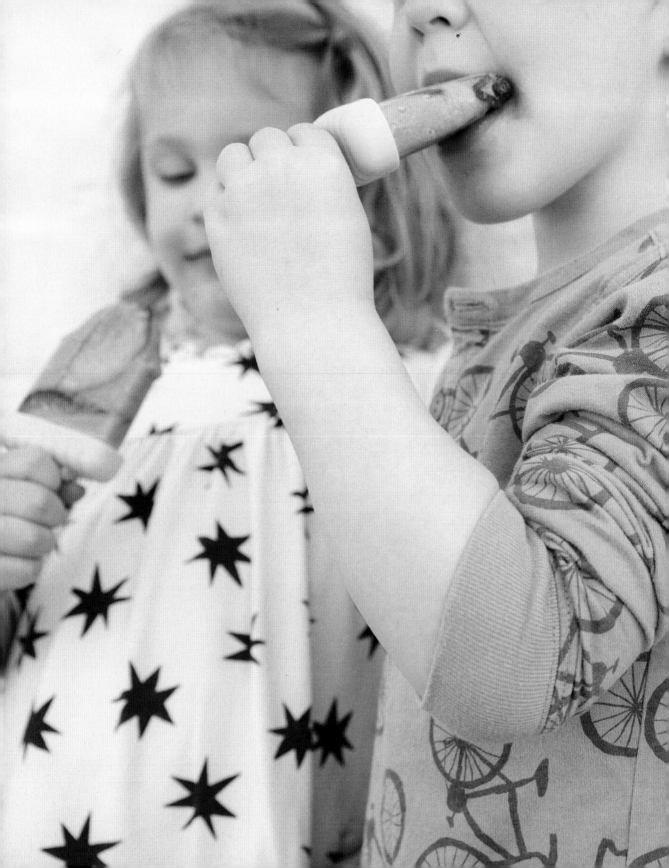

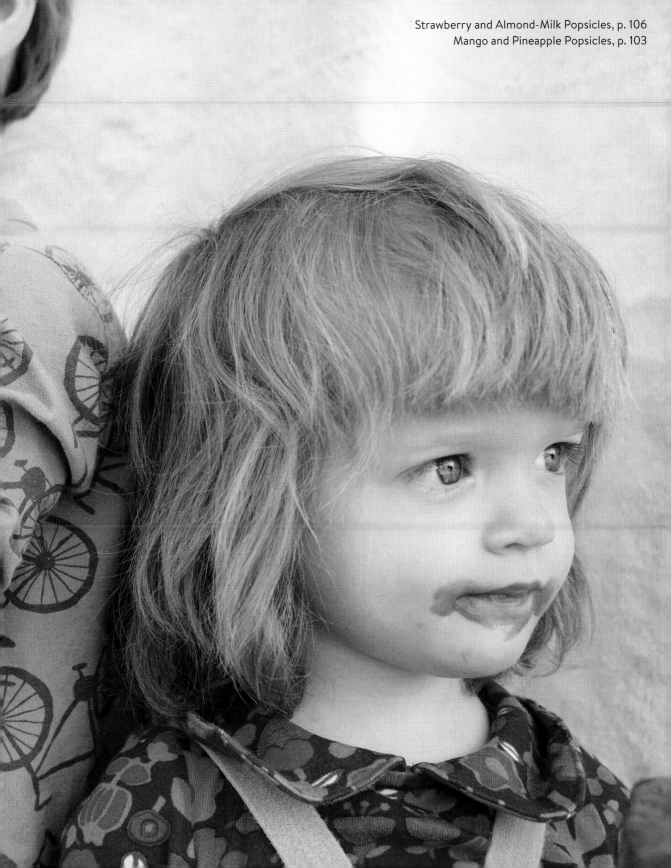

Strawberry and Almond-Milk Popsicles, p. 106
Mango and Pineapple Popsicles, p. 103

2 cups (about
12 medium) hulled
strawberries, divided
1 cup Almond Milk
(page 269)
2 tablespoons maple
syrup
½ teaspoon vanilla
extract
1 small peach, thinly
sliced
¼ cup fresh
blueberries,
preferably wild

Strawberry and Almond–Milk Popsicles

Children see brightly colored ice pops and scream for joy. But the abundance of sugar, artificial colorings, and preservatives can cause a variety of side effects, from allergic reactions to hyperactivity. You won't have to worry about that with these ice pops, which are a healthy crowd-pleaser with both kids and adults.

Thinly slice ½ cup of the strawberries and set aside.

Place the remaining 1½ cups strawberries, almond milk, maple syrup, and vanilla in a blender and blend until smooth and creamy.

Press one or two strawberry and peach slices inside 6 ice-pop molds (see Note). Divide the blueberries among the molds. Pour the strawberry mixture into the molds, being careful not to overfill. Insert the sticks/tops and freeze overnight before serving.

NOTE: I use an ice-pop mold with 6 compartments. You can use whatever size you like, but note that the fill and yield amount may be different. If you don't have an ice-pop mold, use 3- to 5-ounce paper cups. Fill the cups with the mixture, then cover each with foil, cut a slit in the center, and insert a wooden ice-pop stick. Freeze on a tray.

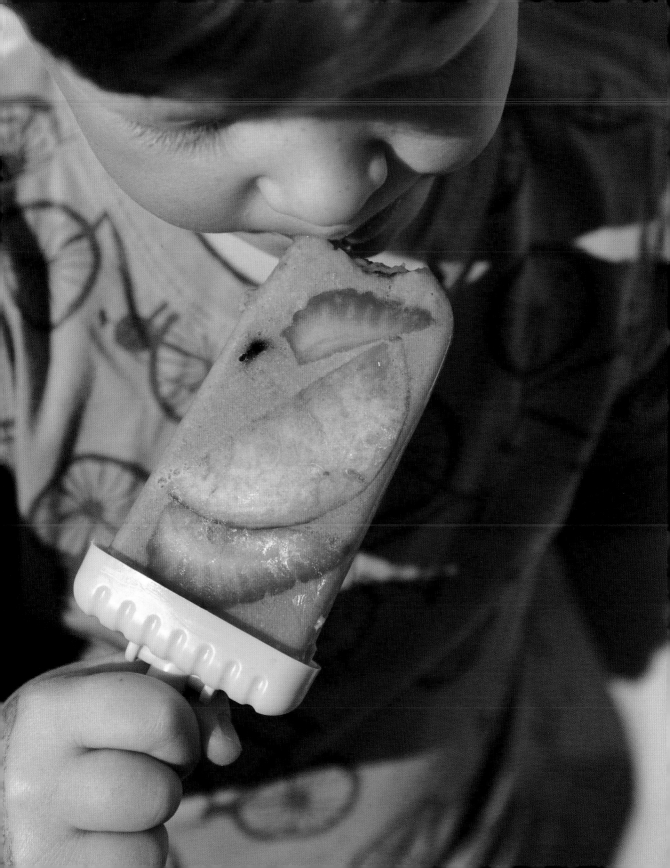

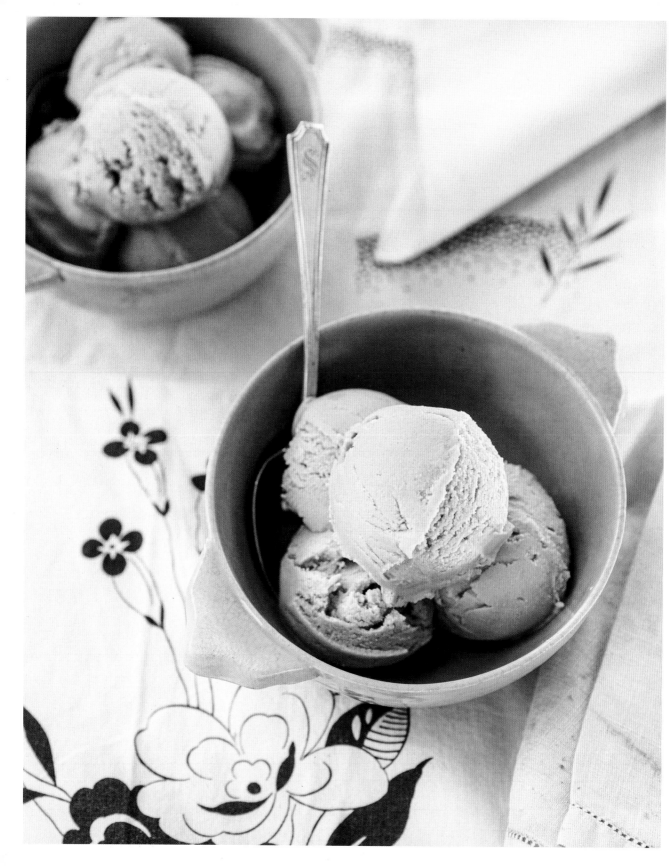

¾ cup raw cashews
¾ cup warm hibiscus
tea
¼ cup melted coconut
oil
1 cup Cashew Milk
(page 273)
1 cup pure maple
syrup
¼ cup peanut oil
1 teaspoon vanilla
extract
½ teaspoon sea salt

Hibiscus and Cashew Ice Cream

Suffice it to say, commercial dairy-free ice creams often have labels
that read like a science project, with ingredients no one can pronounce
and a number of thickeners, such as guar gum and locust bean gum.
Furthermore, they are commonly made with commercial nut milk,
which can be mostly water. This recipe is an easy and tasty alternative
to all of that, plus it doesn't contain any white sugar. I think you'll enjoy
it whether or not you are dairy-free!

The day before you make the ice cream, place the bowl of your ice cream
maker in the freezer.

Soak the cashews in 2 cups water at room temperature for at least
8 hours.

Drain the cashews, discarding the liquid, and place them in a blender
with the tea and coconut oil. Blend until creamy, then add the cashew
milk, maple syrup, peanut oil, vanilla, and salt and continue blending
until thoroughly combined.

If the mixture feels warm to the touch after blending, simply
place the blender in the refrigerator for 15 to 30 minutes or just until
cold to the touch before pouring into your prepared ice cream maker.
Process following the manufacturer's instructions. Serve the ice cream
immediately in its soft-serve stage or transfer it to an airtight freezer-
friendly container and freeze to set completely, about 4 hours.

NOTE: If you do not have an ice cream maker, add the chilled mixture to a
freezer-safe container and freeze. Once every 30 minutes, stir or whisk to
incorporate air. Repeat until almost firm for 6 to 8 hours, then continue
freezing until completely firm. The ice cream won't be as creamy, but it should
still be good.

1 pound strawberries, hulled and sliced
½ cup raw honey (see Notes)
1 teaspoon fresh lemon juice
1½ cups heavy whipping cream
½ cup whole milk
1 teaspoon vanilla extract
⅛ teaspoon sea salt
2 large egg yolks

Strawberry Ice Cream

I have a weakness for ice cream, which is why I created this recipe. It's creamy and satisfying without all the unnecessary additives and preservatives that come with regular store-bought ice cream. Take a scoop—or three!—of this strawberry, honey, and lemon-flavored goodness, and indulge healthfully. If you are lucky enough like me to have access to raw cream and milk, try using it; the result will be even better!

The day before you make the ice cream, place the bowl of your ice cream maker in the freezer.

The next day, in a large bowl, stir together the strawberries, honey, and lemon juice and let macerate for about 20 minutes.

Mash the mixture with a fork, then add the cream, milk, vanilla, salt, and egg yolks and gently stir together. Pour the mixture into the prepared ice cream maker and process following the manufacturer's instructions. Serve the ice cream immediately in its soft-serve stage or transfer it to an airtight freezer-friendly container and freeze to set completely, about 4 hours.

NOTES: Do not serve raw honey to babies twelve months or younger as it may cause infant botulism. Use maple syrup instead.

If you do not have an ice cream maker, add the chilled mixture to a freezer-safe container and freeze. Once every hour, stir or whisk to incorporate air. Repeat until almost firm for 6 to 8 hours, then continue freezing until completely firm. The ice cream won't be as creamy, but it should still be good.

3 cups Coconut
   Milk (page 270) or
   2 (13½-ounce) cans
   full-fat coconut milk
⅓ cup unsweetened
   shredded coconut
¼ cup fresh lime juice
1 tablespoon maple
   syrup
1 teaspoon vanilla
   extract
1 cup diced fresh
   pineapple (½-inch
   pieces)
1 large banana, halved
Toasted shredded
   coconut, for topping
   (optional)

Tropical Vanilla Ice Cream

Coconut ice cream tastes like sunshine in my mouth and reminds me so much of my childhood. I have so many fun memories of sitting under the coconut tree for shade from the blazing sun while praying I didn't get hit on the head with a falling coconut, and of buying coconut sweets from street vendors, not to mention Coconut Jollof Rice (page 189) on Sundays at home, or grandmama's roasted coconut and soaked cassava we ravished at her house. Knowing that coconut is highly nutritive is an added bonus: It is high in protein, fiber, and minerals including manganese, which is essential for bone health and the metabolism of carbohydrates, protein, and cholesterol. This ice cream is delightful even when you are not allergic to dairy!

The day before you make the ice cream, place the bowl of your ice cream maker in the freezer.

Place all the ingredients except the toasted coconut in a high-speed blender and blend until almost smooth; it should still have a little texture from the coconut. Cover and refrigerate for 1 hour.

Pour the mixture into the prepared ice cream maker and process following the manufacturer's instructions. Serve the ice cream immediately in its soft-serve stage or transfer it to an airtight freezer-friendly container and freeze to set completely, about 4 hours.

NOTE: If you do not have an ice cream maker, add the chilled mixture to a freezer-safe container and freeze. Once every hour, stir or whisk to incorporate air. Repeat until almost firm for 6 to 8 hours, then continue freezing until completely firm. The ice cream won't be as creamy, but it should still be good.

Carrot and Zucchini Muffins

3 cups whole wheat pastry flour
½ cup sugar, preferably coconut or date sugar
2¼ teaspoons baking soda
2 teaspoons ground cinnamon
1 teaspoon baking powder
1 teaspoon freshly grated nutmeg
½ teaspoon sea salt
4 large eggs
½ cup melted coconut oil or unsalted butter
2 teaspoons vanilla extract
3 cups grated carrots
2 cups grated zucchini
3 very ripe bananas, mashed (about 1½ cups)

I created this irresistible muffin for a client whose child was an ultra-finicky eater (understatement of the year) and wouldn't touch a vegetable. Suffice it to say, it was a big hit. The carrots and zucchini lend sweetness, flavor, and texture without calling too much attention to themselves. It surprised the heck out of him when he found out what was in the muffins, but in a good way! It was a big step forward for him and his parents. I am generally not a believer of sneaking vegetables into a kid's diet because I feel it's important to help children develop a fondness for foods that they are having difficulty with in an honest way. This applies to adults, too! These muffins are delicious, no matter who you are sharing them with.

Preheat the oven to 350°F. Line 2 standard 12-cup muffin pans with cupcake liners.

In a medium bowl, whisk together the flour, sugar, baking soda, cinnamon, baking powder, nutmeg, and salt. In a large bowl, whisk together the eggs, oil or butter, and vanilla, then add the carrots, zucchini, and bananas and mix well. Add the dry ingredients to the wet ingredients and gently fold together, being careful not to overmix.

Spoon the batter into the prepared muffin pans and bake until a toothpick inserted into the center comes out clean, 25 to 30 minutes. Remove from the oven and let set for 10 minutes, then transfer from the pans to a wire rack and let cool completely. Serve, then store any leftovers, which can be frozen for up to 3 months in an airtight container. (Yep, that is going to be difficult because your home will smell like a beautiful fall morning, but try as best as you can.)

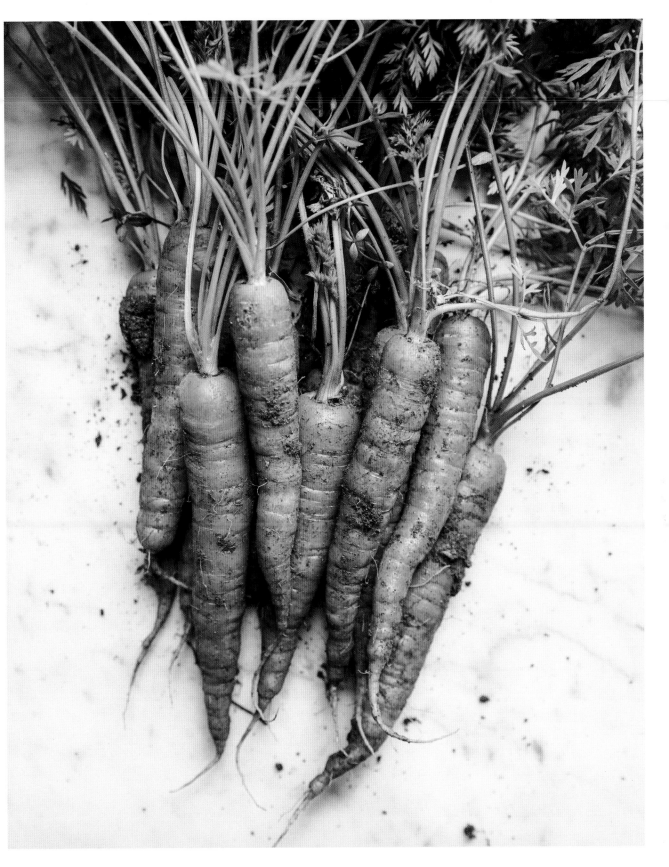

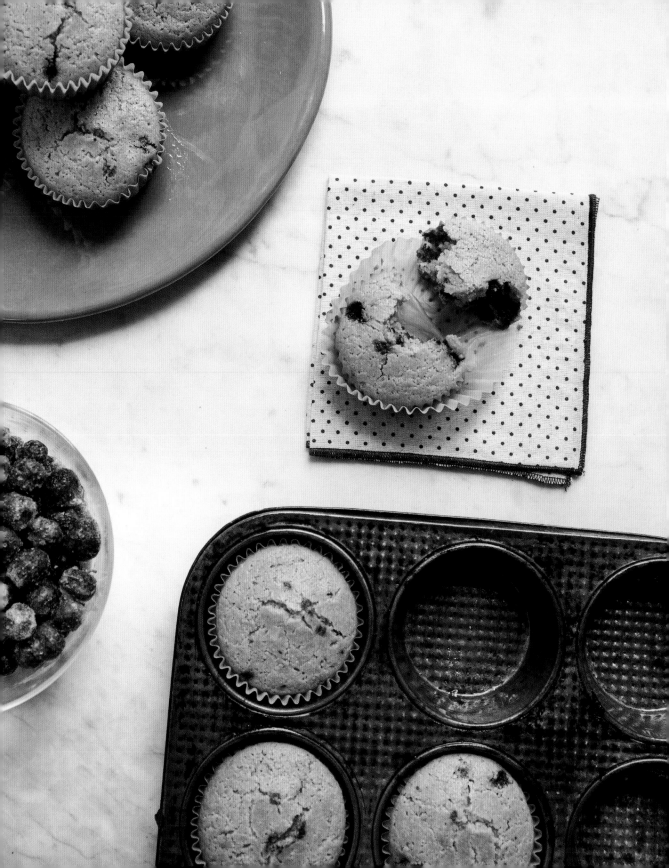

1 cup cornmeal
1 cup quinoa flour
2 tablespoons baking
  powder
½ teaspoon sea salt
¼ cup melted coconut
  oil
⅓ cup raw honey (see
  Note)
1 cup Coconut Milk
  (page 270)
2 large eggs
½ teaspoon
  vanilla extract
Zest of 1 lemon
1 cup fresh or
  frozen blueberries,
  preferably wild

Gluten-Free, Dairy-Free Quinoa-Blueberry Muffins

Looking for a quick and easy gluten-free muffin? The grocery store aisles are full of options but, unfortunately, many of the commercial gluten-free baked goods are filled with highly refined carbohydrates and modified starches, artificial sugars, inflammatory omega-6 vegetable oils, food dyes, food stabilizers, and gums. Well, this muffin has none of that—it is full of essential micronutrients and contains zero dairy. All that and it tastes incredible, too!

Preheat the oven to 400°F. Line a standard 12-cup muffin pan with cupcake liners.

Sift together the cornmeal, quinoa flour, baking powder, and salt into a large bowl. In a medium bowl, whisk together the cocount oil and honey until smooth, then whisk in the coconut milk, eggs, vanilla, and zest. Add the wet ingredients to the dry ingredients and mix. Fold in the blueberries, being careful not to overmix.

Spoon the batter into the prepared muffin pan and bake until a toothpick inserted into the center comes out clean, 15 to 20 minutes. Let cool for about 5 minutes before removing from the pan. If storing for later, let the muffins cool completely. They can be frozen for up to 3 months in an airtight container. These are best served warm.

NOTE: Do not serve raw honey to babies twelve months or younger, as it may cause infant botulism. Use maple syrup instead.

Spinach and Thyme Cheese Straws

I love cheese straws as much as the next person, especially when they are embellished with slivers of baby spinach and fresh thyme. Those additions don't just lend flavor and color—they lend health benefits, too. Spinach is full of vitamin K, and thyme is known for its anti-inflammatory, antimicrobial, and antioxidant properties. Bonus: The cheese straws are a snap to make thanks to store-bought puff pastry.

Preheat the oven to 375°F. Line a baking sheet with parchment paper.

In a small bowl, stir together the spinach, cheese, and thyme.

Lightly flour a clean work surface, unfold the pastry, lightly dust a rolling pin with flour, and gently roll the puff pastry, 3 or 4 times to get it a little flat. Brush the puff pastry with the beaten egg wash, then sprinkle evenly with the spinach mixture.

Using a pizza cutter or sharp knife, cut the pastry into 12 strips. Fold each strip lengthwise so the spinach mixture is on the inside. Working with one strip at a time, twist the two ends in opposite directions several times, then place on the prepared baking sheet, spacing the strips about 1 inch apart.

Bake for about 15 minutes, then flip the sticks and bake until golden brown, about 5 minutes more. Let cool for at least 5 minutes before serving.

1 cup thinly sliced baby spinach

¼ cup freshly grated Parmesan cheese, preferably Parmigiano Reggiano

1 teaspoon fresh thyme leaves

All-purpose flour, for rolling out the dough

1 sheet puff pastry, thawed

1 large egg, beaten with 1 tablespoon water

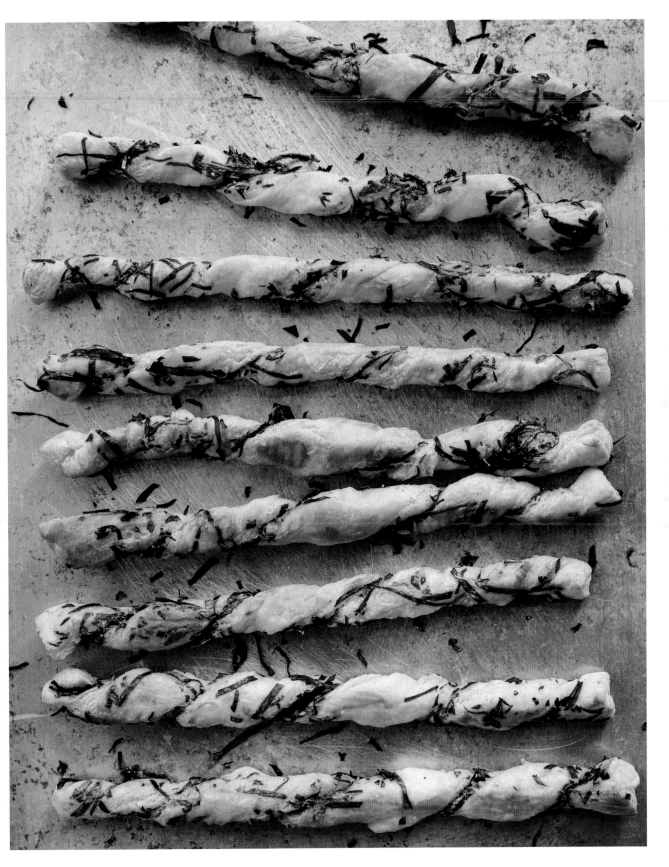

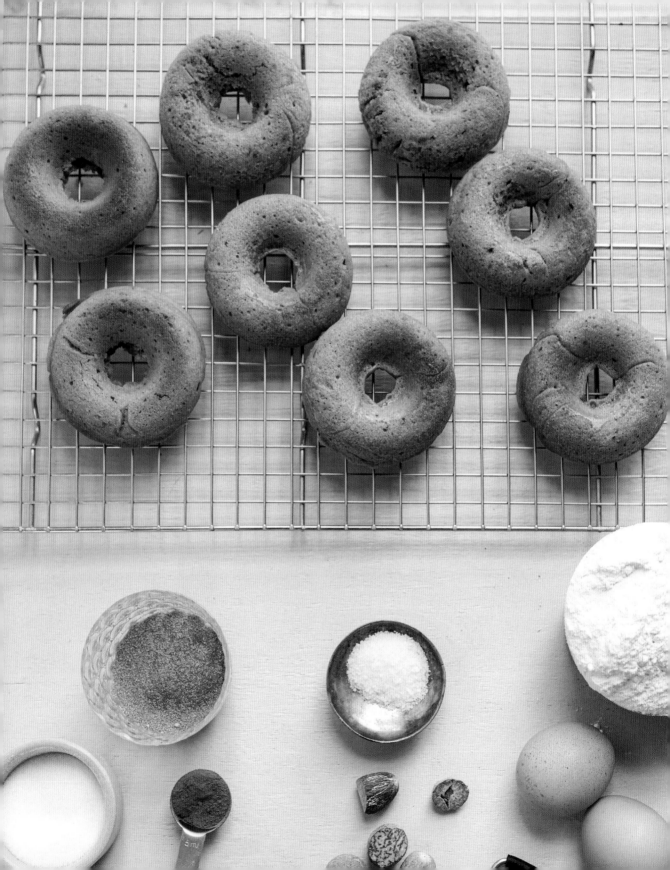

Baked Sweet Potato Doughnuts

¼ cup coconut oil, plus
more for greasing
the pan
2 large eggs
¾ cup sweet potato
puree (see Note)
⅓ cup plus
3 tablespoons sugar
1 tablespoon ground
cinnamon, divided
1 teaspoon baking
powder
1 teaspoon freshly
grated nutmeg
½ teaspoon sea salt
1 cup whole wheat
pastry flour

These doughnuts are a healthy twist to the classic fried version, but are still a favorite treat in my house and with my clients. Not only are they baked, they are made with whole wheat flour and pureed sweet potato, one of the richest natural sources of beta-carotene, a plant-based compound that is converted to vitamin A in the body. Vitamin A is critical to a healthy immune system. Meanwhile, the cinnamon and nutmeg lend healing benefits. And did I mention that the doughnuts are absolutely delicious?

Preheat the oven to 350°F. Grease a standard 6-cavity doughnut pan lightly with coconut oil and set aside.

In a large bowl, mix together the coconut oil, eggs, sweet potato puree, ⅓ cup sugar, 1 teaspoon of the cinnamon, the baking powder, nutmeg, and salt until combined. Stir in the flour and continue to mix until smooth.

Fill the wells of the prepared doughnut pan about three-quarters full. Bake the doughnuts until golden, 15 to 17 minutes. Let cool for about 5 minutes.

Meanwhile, in a large plastic bag, combine the remaining 3 tablespoons of sugar and the remaining 2 teaspoons of cinnamon. Place the doughnuts in the bag one at a time and shake lightly to coat. Serve warm or at room temperature.

NOTE: To make sweet potato puree, steam 1 medium sweet potato for about 30 minutes, then peel, puree, and cool.

Carroty Cake Balls

When your sweet tooth is in overdrive, look no further. These super-delicious and healthy treats, made with carrots, dates, coconut, and a smidgen of cardamom, are sure to satisfy. The only problem is that it's hard to stop eating them, so consider making an extra batch! They freeze well, too.

¾ cup unsweetened shredded coconut, divided
6 Medjool dates, pitted and finely chopped
¾ cup walnuts, roughly chopped
½ cup grated carrots
¼ cup hemp seeds
3 tablespoons raw honey (see Note)
1 teaspoon vanilla extract
½ teaspoon freshly grated nutmeg
¼ teaspoon ground cardamon
¼ teaspoon sea salt

Line a sheet pan with parchment paper and set aside. Place ¼ cup of the coconut on a plate and set aside. Place the dates, remaining ½ cup of the coconut, walnuts, carrots, hemp seeds, honey, vanilla, nutmeg, cardamom, and salt in a food processor and pulse until a sticky "dough" forms.

Form the mixture into about 15 (1-inch) balls. Roll the balls in the coconut until completely covered and transfer to the prepared sheet pan. Refrigerate, covered, for at least 4 hours, then serve either cold or at room temperature.

NOTE: Do not serve raw honey to babies twelve months or younger, as it may cause infant botulism. Use maple syrup instead.

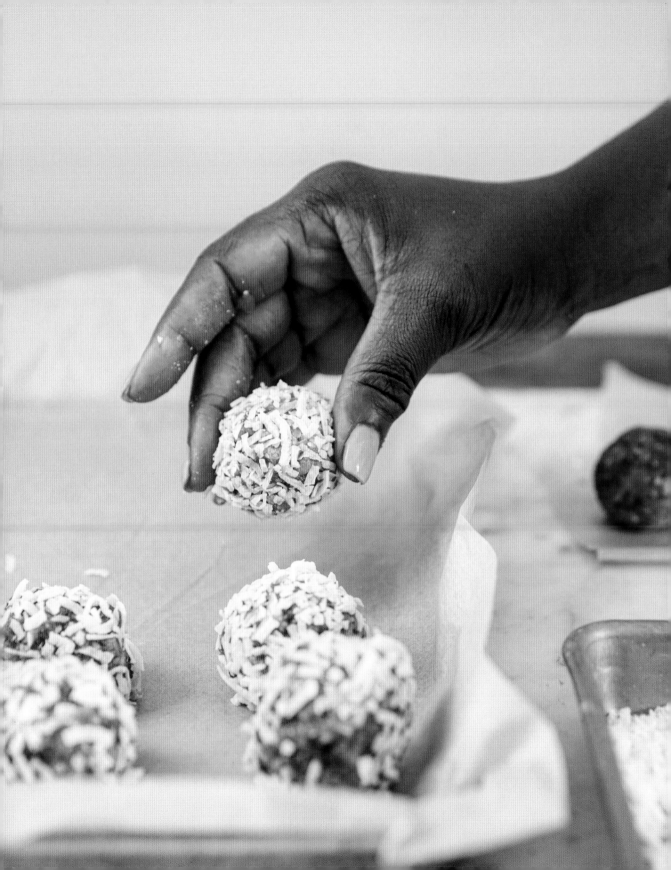

Buttery Pound Cake

SERVES 8 TO 12

3 sticks butter, plus more for greasing the pan
3 cups all-purpose flour, plus more for dusting the pan
1 cup sugar
5 large eggs, at room temperature
1 teaspoon freshly grated nutmeg
½ teaspoon baking powder
½ teaspoon sea salt
1 cup whole milk
1 teaspoon vanilla extract

I made my very first cake at age nine, and my mami loved it so much that I quickly became the family baker. When I moved to the United States in my early twenties, I was so excited when I saw pound cake at the grocery store. We didn't have that in Cameroon or Nigeria when I was growing up, and it looked so fancy and fluffy. As soon as I got home, I excitedly cut a big slice and took a bite, which I immediately spit out. I had never tasted anything so sweet in my life. When I looked at the label, I was shocked and confused that it listed more than 20 ingredients, many with words I'd never heard of. This recipe is the antithesis of that cake, and a celebration of my childhood baking days.

Preheat the oven to 300°F. Generously grease and flour a 10-inch tube pan, shaking out any excess flour, and set aside.

Cream together the butter and sugar in an electric stand mixer using the paddle attachment, (you can also use an electric hand mixer) on high speed for about 8 minutes or until very light and fluffy. Reduce the speed to medium and add the eggs one at a time, beating in each for about a minute before adding the next one. Scrape the sides of the bowl with a spatula as needed.

In a medium bowl, gently stir together the flour, nutmeg, baking powder, and salt. In a small bowl (or the measuring cup used to measure the milk), stir together the milk and vanilla.

With the mixer on medium speed, add the dry ingredients to the butter mixture about a ½ cup at a time, alternating with a little of the milk, and ending with the flour mixture. Scrape down the sides and bottom of the bowl and mix again on medium speed until well combined, a few minutes more.

Pour the batter into the prepared pan and bake until a toothpick inserted in the center comes out clean, about 1½ hours. Let the cake cool for at least 20 minutes, then carefully invert it onto a rack to cool completely before serving. Can be frozen for up to 6 months in an airtight container.

NOTE: You can make this dairy-free using Cashew Milk (page 273). The cake will be a little dense but will taste just as delicious.

¼ cup pitted and chopped Medjool dates
¼ packed cup dried cherries
¼ cup goji berries
¼ cup chopped roasted pistachios
¼ cup sesame seeds
1 tablespoon unsweetened shredded coconut
9 ounces dark (60 to 70 percent cacao) chocolate, chopped and melted (see Notes)

Dark–Chocolate Coins

We had a few cacao trees at the back of our home growing up. After we would harvest the pods that Mami would let us have, we would spend time sucking the juicy flesh of the beans. We would then dry the beans for days for cacao nibs, which would be ground into powder. That bitter crunch of cacao nibs is still my favorite way to experience pure joy. Looking back, I can now understand why we were always so full of energy. Cacao has so many amazing health benefits, including the highest plant-based source of iron, high in antioxidants, calcium, and more. It is also a great source of four feel-good chemicals: serotonin, tryptophan, tyrosine, and phenylethylamine, which are associated with cozy feelings of well-being and happiness and can even alleviate depression. These coins are a true health food!

Line a baking sheet with parchment paper and set aside.

In a small bowl, stir together the dates, cherries, goji berries, pistachios, sesame seeds, and coconut and set aside.

Using a 1-tablespoon measuring spoon, scoop melted chocolate onto the prepared baking sheet and carefully spread using the back of the spoon to create even 2-inch circles. Sprinkle the date mixture evenly over each circle as you go, then refrigerate until hardened, about 30 minutes. Serve.

Store any leftovers in an airtight container in the refrigerator, separated by parchment paper.

NOTES: Using a high-quality semi-sweet chocolate with 60 to 70 percent cacao will yield the tastiest results.

If you want smaller coins, use a teaspoon to scoop chocolate; you'll have about 30 coins.

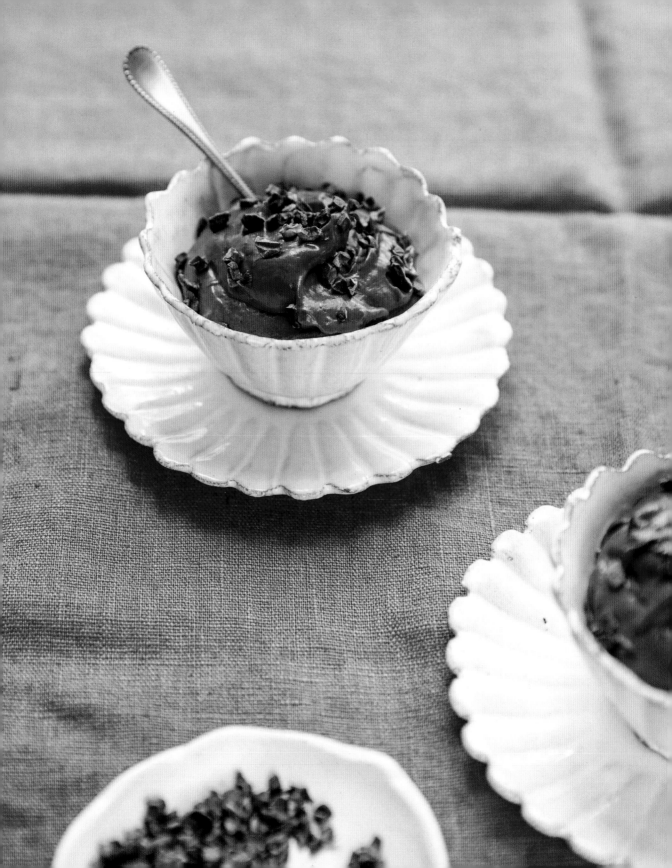

Turmeric and Chocolate Mousse

GF, DF

SERVES 6 TO 8

1 cup Almond Milk
(page 269)
6 Medjool dates, pitted
1 ripe avocado, halved,
pitted, and peeled
¼ cup cocoa powder,
at least 70 percent
cacao
2 tablespoons freshly
squeezed orange
juice
½ teaspoon chia
powder
¼ teaspoon ground
turmeric
1 tablespoon maple
syrup, or to taste
1 tablespoon grated
orange zest
(optional)
Toppings of choice
(chocolate
shavings, cacao
nibs, raspberries,
blackberries, etc.;
optional)

Chocolate mousse gets a healthy makeover here without sacrificing the creamy, light, deep chocolate flavor we love about the treat. Avocado, dates, almond milk, and magnesium-rich cocoa powder form the base, which is enhanced by orange and ground turmeric. The turmeric's active ingredient, curcumin, has powerful anti-inflammatory and antioxidant properties that help protect us from disease and premature aging. The best part is that when I serve the mousse, most people never guess that it's missing the typical cream, eggs, and butter!

In a small saucepan, warm the almond milk over medium heat, then remove from the heat and add the dates. Soak until plump, about 30 minutes.

In a high-speed blender, puree the dates with just enough of the almond milk (start with ½ cup) as needed to get a creamy paste. Add the avocado and blend until smooth and creamy. Add the cocoa powder, orange juice, chia powder, and turmeric and blend until you get a smooth mousse-like texture, adding a little more almond milk, if needed.

Taste and adjust the sweetness with maple syrup, if needed. Transfer to a container, stir in the orange zest, if using, and chill, covered, for at least 30 minutes.

To serve, spoon or pipe the mousse into small bowls or ramekins and garnish with toppings of choice, if using.

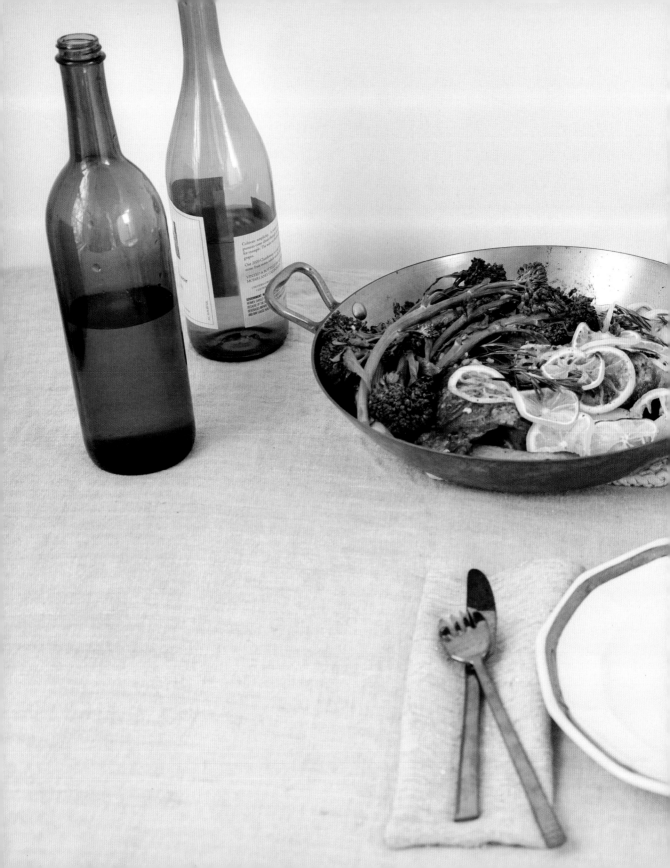

Mains | MEAT

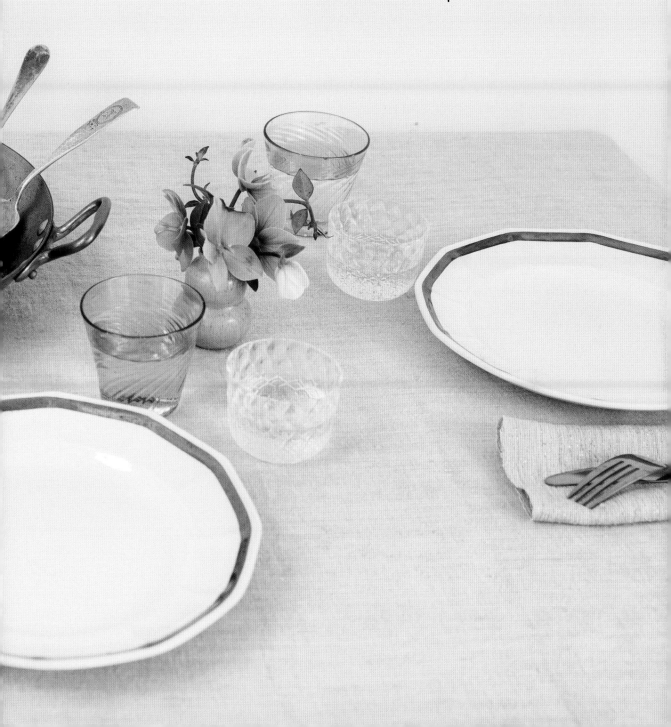

THE MODERN DIET DILEMMA: IS IT
better to eat meat or go vegan or
something in between? Some people
believe meat consumption causes cancer and is
damaging to the planet; others argue that it's
important to eat meat for nutritional reasons.
People on both sides of the conversation
tend to be judgmental, so much so that these
conversations can be very difficult to listen to.

The truth is, humans around the world
have been eating meat or only plants and
thriving for centuries. For me, the issue we
should be focusing on is not vegan versus non-
vegan (those are very personal preferences and
no one should be vilified for their choice), but
rather the quality of the meat that is readily
available to those who want it.

Good meat is nourishing. For proof, look
to the Maasai people in Kenya and northern
Tanzania. They eat raw meat regularly and
on special occasions even drink cow's blood,
yet they have a much lower incidence of
disease compared to Americans and boast an
unusually high number of centenarians.

The problem in the U.S. is that factory
farming has flooded the market with
inexpensive meat (and dairy) products that
have substantially contributed to the ever-
growing cases of chronic diseases. Livestock
are fed the cheapest food to fatten them up,
which lowers the quality and nutritional value
of their meat and milk, while increasing our
resistance to antibiotics and polluting the air,
land, and water. Yes, factory farming enables
us to have plenty of cheap meat and dairy, but
at what cost?

By contrast, according to a recent
Compassion in World Farming report, meat
and dairy from pasture-raised animals are the
total opposite of factory farms; these animals
are raised in open pastures, eating the diet
(grass) they are designed to eat. The truth is
that, like humans, animals that eat the proper
diet—one that's geared toward their unique
digestive systems—and that are given room
to roam in open pasture, exercise, and play
as nature intended stay healthy and strong
throughout their entire lives without need
of antibiotics. Because they are allowed to
gain weight naturally and mature as nature
intended without supplement, rather than
being forced to gain weight at an unnatural
rate with growth hormones, their meat often
contains higher levels of antioxidants and iron,
lower levels of fat, and two to four times more
of the healthy omega-3 fatty acids and better
ratios of omega-3 to omega-6 fatty acids.

When I was growing up in Cameroon all
our meat was grass-fed and pasture-raised.
When I moved to the United States in 1990

GENERAL MEAT TIPS

When possible, I prefer to cook meat on the bone, just like my mami taught me. Bones are a good source of various minerals, collagen (called gelatin once cooked), and amino acids. "Collagen" literally comes from the Greek word for "glue" and is what holds our bones together. Our bodies need both collagen and amino acids as building blocks for our own collagen production and many other critical functions. Our bodies also use minerals for carrying oxygen, enzyme function, hormone health, and bone health. Since we cannot create minerals, we must obtain them from food.

Cooking with bones provides a simple, delicious, and inexpensive way to receive all those key benefits.

Switching to pasture-raised chickens may be better for your health, but it can also make you happier—literally. Compared to their mass-produced cousins, pasture-raised birds have higher levels of tryptophan, an essential amino acid that can boost serotonin, which has been linked to feelings of improved well-being. Bonus: Their skin is healthier, too, so if you've been avoiding chicken skin because it's "bad" for you, feel free to indulge!

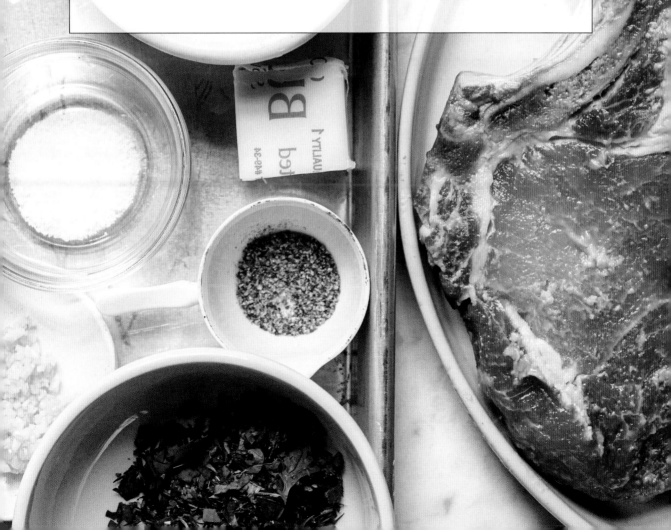

I realized that meat in America didn't taste as good as meat at home. Not only are pasture-raised meat and dairy better for your health, better for the animals, better for the environment, and better for the farmer, but they also taste better than conventionally raised meat and dairy products.

My advice is, if you're going to eat meat, try to get the good stuff, even if it means having to pay a bit more or buy less. Choose meat labeled "pasture-raised" and "grass-fed"; if money is not an issue add "organic" to the list to ensure you're getting the safest, most nutritious options similar to what our ancestors consumed before us. You can generally find pasture-raised meat everywhere, including at warehouse retailers, large grocery stores, farmers markets, health food stores, and food cooperatives. Find a local farm in your area. You might actually find it is part of a community-sponsored agriculture (CSA) drop, making it possible for you to buy directly from the farmer.

Once you buy your meat, use it in whatever recipes in this section appeal to you. They are all dishes I make regularly for my own family and my clients, with an emphasis on healthfulness and flavor. I am a time-strapped mama, and while I love and appreciate the slow days when we all sit together having beautiful conversations while I cook nourishing meals for the family, my reality on most days is far from this. Life gets really hectic, and I turn to simple meals that can be pulled together quickly, like my Sheet Pan Flank Steak with Carrots and Potatoes (page 147), or extended for days, like my Beef and Butternut Squash Chili with Beans (page 131). This is the ultimate multipurpose meal—we never get bored with it since there are a zillion ways to serve it. Day one we eat it with rice or a good slice of sourdough bread. Day two it is wrapped in a tortilla with a sprinkle of cheese and sizzled on the skillet. For an entirely different experience, on day three, I serve the chili with sweet plantains with scoops of salsa and a side salad. One dish gives three days' worth of meals! For days that I still want to cook but want time to put my feet up after a long day at work I love my One-Skillet, Date-Night Lemony Chicken (page 158). As you begin to cook through the recipes, my hope is you, too, will find your favorites.

Beef and Butternut Squash Chili with Beans

A big pot of hearty chili is always satisfying. To make this version extra nourishing, I add squash to increase the fiber content, which is key to good gut health. The dish is filling and delicious as is, but you can also serve it with your favorite toppings. If you like, you can prepare this in a slow cooker. After cooking the meat, combine all the ingredients in your slow cooker, cover, and cook on low for 4 to 6 hours.

In a large pot, heat the oil over medium-high heat. Add the onion and cook, stirring occasionally, until translucent, about 5 minutes. Add the garlic and cook, stirring, for about 1 minute.

Add the ground beef and cook, breaking it up with a wooden spoon and stirring occasionally, until no longer pink, 5 to 7 minutes. If there's an excessive amount of grease, drain some of it. Stir in the spices, salt, and bell peppers and cook, stirring occasionally, for about 5 minutes more.

Stir in the squash, beans, tomatoes, and broth and cook, covered, over low heat, stirring occasionally, for about 30 minutes.

Serve in individual bowls.

3 tablespoons olive oil
1 large onion, chopped
2 cloves garlic, minced
2 pounds ground beef
2 teaspoons ground cumin
2 teaspoons dried oregano
2 teaspoons pumpkin spice
1 teaspoon chili powder
1 teaspoon smoked paprika
1 teaspoon sea salt
1 large red bell pepper, seeded and diced
1 large yellow bell pepper, seeded and diced
4 cups 1-inch cubed butternut squash (from about 1 small butternut squash)
3 cups cooked black beans, drained; if using canned, drained and rinsed
3 cups diced tomatoes or diced or crushed canned tomatoes, undrained
2 cups low-sodium beef broth

Meatloaf with Vegetables

I am a firm believer that every meal is an opportunity to nourish the body any little way you can without it feeling like chaos. Here, I take the basic meatloaf dish and boost its health benefits by adding fiber-rich carrot and celery, scallions for their anti-inflammatory benefit and extra dose of vitamin C. Whether you are feeding children or adults (or both!), especially that picky eater for whom every bite is a labor of love, you feel good knowing you got a little extra dose of nourishment in your favorite meatloaf. You can enjoy the meatloaf on a bed of my delicious Kale Salad (page 249) or Mashed Potatoes (page 143).

Preheat the oven to 350°F. Grease a 9 × 5–inch loaf pan with olive oil and set aside.

In a large skillet, heat the oil over medium heat. Add the onion and cook, stirring occasionally, until translucent, about 5 minutes. Add the carrot, celery, salt, and pepper and cook, stirring occasionally, until the vegetables are just tender, about 5 minutes more. Add the garlic, scallions, and thyme and cook, stirring, for 1 minute. Stir in the tomato paste and Worcestershire sauce, then set aside and let cool.

In a large bowl, whisk the eggs. Add the cooled vegetables and bread crumbs and mix well. Add the ground beef and gently mix. (Do not overmix or the meatloaf will be rubbery.) Scoop the mixture into the prepared pan and gently press it into the pan.

Brush the top of the meatloaf with half of the ketchup and bake for 45 minutes. Brush with the remaining ketchup and bake until the middle of the loaf reaches 155°F on a meat thermometer, 15 to 20 minutes. Let cool for about 15 minutes before slicing and serving.

1 tablespoon olive oil, plus more for greasing the pan
1 onion, finely chopped
1 carrot, finely chopped
1 stalk celery, finely chopped
1½ teaspoons sea salt
1 teaspoon freshly ground black pepper
2 cloves garlic, minced
4 scallions, finely chopped
1 teaspoon chopped fresh thyme leaves
1 tablespoon tomato paste
1 teaspoon Worcestershire sauce
2 large eggs
½ cup bread crumbs
2 pounds ground beef
½ cup ketchup

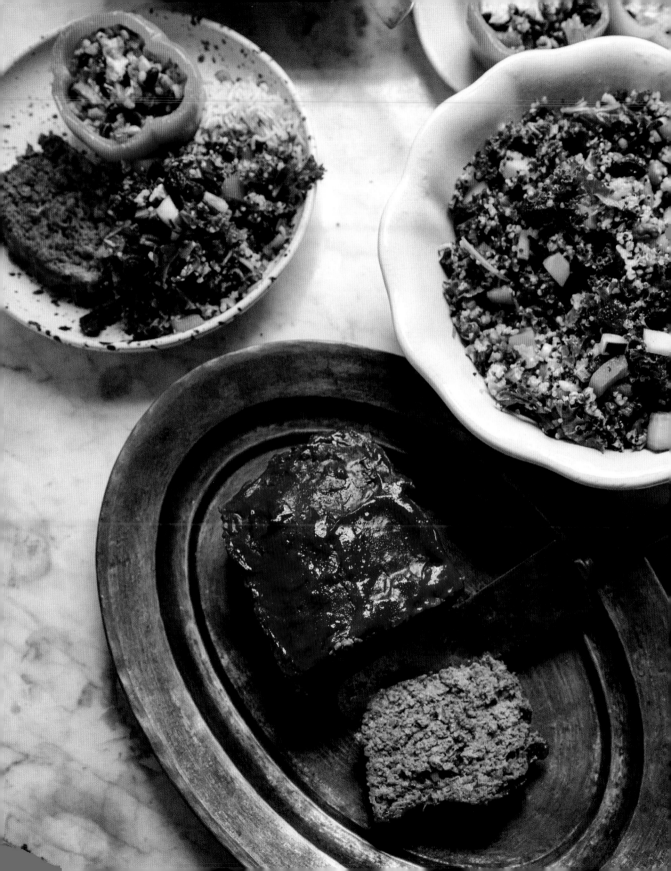

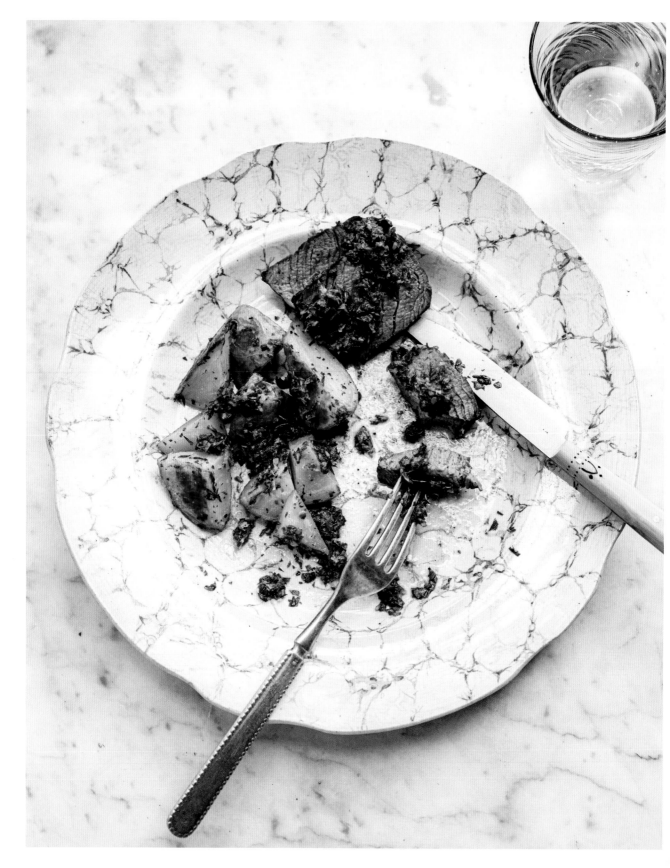

Beef Tenderloin with Rosemary and Thyme Potatoes

Pairing beef tenderloin with roasted skin-on potatoes and a refreshing basil sauce adds to the nutritional value of this dish. Potatoes often get a bad rap, but did you know that eating the potato skin will provide more fiber, vitamins, minerals, and phytochemicals than eating just the flesh? Rosemary and thyme are two of my favorite herbs. Not only are they incredibly flavorful, fragrant, and versatile, but they are also nutritional powerhouses filled with antioxidants and anti-inflammatory compounds, which are thought to help boost the immune system and improve blood circulation. This dish is easy, but impressive enough for any guests, including the in-laws.

Preheat the oven to 425°F. Line a sheet pan with parchment paper.

For the potatoes, in a large bowl, toss together all the ingredients, transfer to a parchment-lined sheet pan, and bake until tender, golden brown, and crispy, 30 to 35 minutes, tossing after about 20 minutes.

Meanwhile, prepare the sauce. In a small bowl, stir together the parsley, basil, oregano, garlic, 2 tablespoons of the oil, the lemon zest, lemon juice, red pepper flakes, and ¼ teaspoon of salt, or to taste, then set aside.

When the potatoes have about 8 minutes left, prepare the tenderloin steaks. Use 1 teaspoon of the oil to coat the steaks, then sprinkle the meat with ¼ teaspoon salt each, or to taste, and the pepper.

In a large ovenproof skillet, heat the remaining 2 teaspoons of oil over medium-high heat. Add the steaks and cook for 3 minutes on each side for medium-rare, 130°F on a meat thermometer (or less or more, as desired). Allow to rest while the potatoes finish roasting. Transfer to four plates or a platter and serve with the potatoes and sauce. If you don't want to turn on the oven, you can also roast the potatoes using an air fryer at 350°F for 15 minutes, tossing halfway through cooking.

ROASTED POTATOES

1½ pounds unpeeled Yukon gold potatoes, quartered
1 tablespoon olive oil
1 tablespoon finely chopped fresh rosemary leaves
1 tablespoon finely chopped fresh thyme leaves
1 teaspoon onion powder
¼ teaspoon sea salt
¼ teaspoon freshly ground black pepper

TENDERLOIN STEAKS AND SAUCE

¼ cup chopped fresh flat-leaf parsley
3 tablespoons chopped fresh basil
1 teaspoon chopped fresh oregano leaves
3 cloves garlic, minced
3 tablespoons olive oil, divided
½ teaspoon grated lemon zest
1 tablespoon fresh lemon juice
¼ teaspoon crushed red pepper flakes
1¼ teaspoons sea salt, or to taste, divided
4 (4-ounce) beef tenderloin steaks, about 1 inch thick
1 teaspoon freshly ground black pepper

2 tablespoons olive oil, plus more for greasing the pan
1 teaspoon ground cumin
½ teaspoon chili powder, divided
¾ teaspoon sea salt, divided
½ teaspoon freshly ground black pepper
1 large onion, cut into ½-inch-wide slices
2 green bell peppers, cut into ½-inch-wide slices
2 red bell peppers, cut into ½-inch-wide slices
2 yellow bell peppers, cut into ½-inch-wide slices
12 ounces flank steak, thinly sliced
½ cup plain yogurt of choice
1 teaspoon fresh lime juice
1 teaspoon sriracha, or to taste
¼ cup chopped fresh cilantro
1 lime, cut into wedges
8 (6-inch) corn tortillas

Sheet Pan Steak Fajitas

This is one of my back-pocket recipes. It couldn't be quicker or easier and everyone loves it. I set all the components on the table—including a spicy, creamy sauce made with sriracha and yogurt—and people pick and choose what they want, then assemble their own fajitas, I also intentionally make the steak a side show, allowing the vegetables to take center stage; a little slice of succulent meat goes a long way with roasted peppers. Trust me, your family won't miss the large beef portions. The probiotics from the live active cultures in the yogurt also lend more gut-friendly and immunity-boosting nutrients.

Preheat the broiler, with a rack in the top position. Place a sheet pan in the oven while it heats.

In a medium bowl, whisk together the oil, cumin, ¼ teaspoon of chili powder, ½ teaspoon of salt, and the black pepper. Place the onion and bell peppers in a large bowl, add half of the oil mixture and toss to coat. Add the steak to the remaining oil mixture and toss to coat.

Carefully remove the hot sheet pan from the oven and lightly brush it with olive oil to coat. Spread the onion and peppers across the pan and broil until almost tender, about 10 minutes.

Meanwhile, make the spicy sauce. In a small bowl, whisk together the yogurt, lime juice, sriracha, remaining ¼ teaspoon of chili powder— please omit if you don't need the extra kick—and ¼ teaspoon of salt, then set aside.

When the onion and peppers are ready, move them to the sides of the pan, spread the steak out in the center, and broil until the steak reaches the desired degree of doneness, about 3 minutes for medium-rare. Remove from the oven, sprinkle the cilantro over the top, and arrange the lime wedges on the pan.

Heat the tortillas according to the package directions and serve alongside the sheet pan with the sauce.

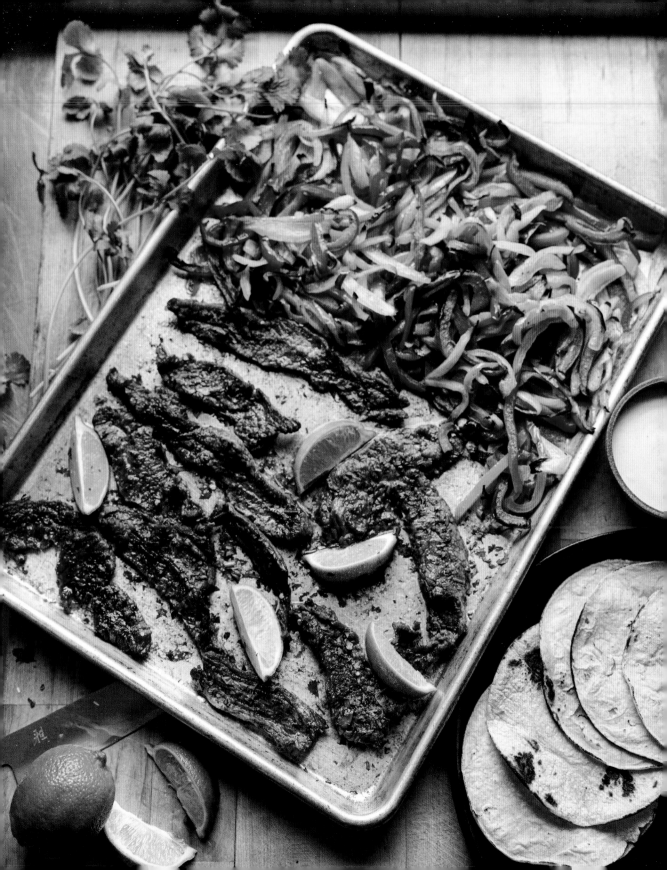

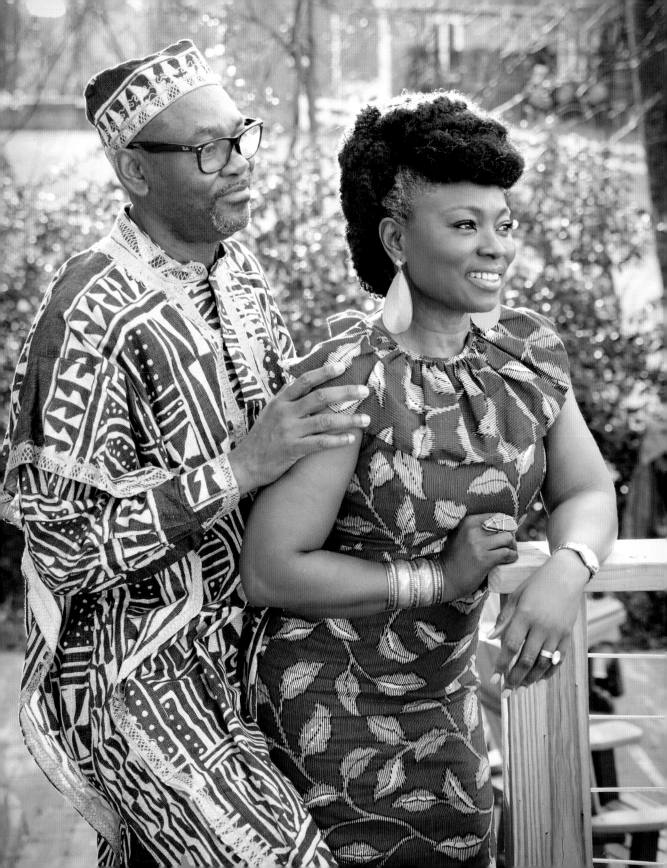

Bolognese Sauce

GF, DF

SERVES 6

This Bolognese sauce will nourish your body with nutrients and your soul with comfort. As a mama I so love the fact that I still get a delicious pot of thick and creamy sauce despite making adjustments to fit our busy lifestyle, and I love the many nutrients in this dish. Celery, for example, offers protection to the entire digestive tract thanks to pectin-based polysaccharides, which have been shown to decrease instances of stomach ulcers and improve the lining of the stomach. Even picky eaters tend to like this sauce. Serve it with pasta or zoodles or in lasagna or pot pie.

2 tablespoons olive oil
1 large onion, finely chopped
4 cloves garlic, minced
3 stalks celery, finely chopped
1 carrot, finely chopped
4 ounces pancetta, finely chopped
1½ pounds ground beef
1 cup low-sodium beef broth
1 cup Cashew Milk (page 273)
1 pound tomatoes, chopped
1 (6-ounce) can tomato paste
½ cup chopped fresh flat-leaf parsley
2 tablespoons chopped fresh thyme leaves
¼ teaspoon crushed red pepper flakes
⅛ teaspoon freshly grated nutmeg
2½ teaspoons sea salt
¼ teaspoon freshly ground black pepper

In a large Dutch oven or pot, heat the oil over medium heat. Add the onion and cook, stirring occasionally, until translucent, about 5 minutes. Add the garlic and cook, stirring, for about 30 seconds. Add the celery and carrot and cook, stirring occasionally, for about 5 minutes more.

Add the pancetta and cook, stirring occasionally, for 5 minutes. Add the beef and cook, breaking up the meat with a wooden spoon and stirring occasionally, until no large chunks or traces of pink remain, about 7 minutes. Spoon off and discard any excess fat.

Stir in the broth, cashew milk, tomatoes, tomato paste, parsley, thyme, red pepper flakes, nutmeg, salt, and black pepper and bring to a simmer over medium heat. Reduce the heat and gently simmer, partially covered, until the meat is tender, about 45 minutes. If storing, allow to cool down completely. Sauce will last for up to 4 days in the refrigerator in an airtight container, and up to 3 months in the freezer.

Grandma's Meatballs

1 large egg
2 pounds ground beef
½ onion, finely chopped
3 cloves garlic, finely chopped
½ cup freshly grated Parmesan cheese, preferably Parmigiano Reggiano
⅓ cup bread crumbs
¼ cup chopped fresh flat-leaf parsley
1 cup finely chopped baby spinach
1½ teaspoons Italian seasoning
1½ teaspoons sea salt
1 teaspoon freshly ground black pepper
¼ cup milk
2 tablespoons olive oil

Our youngest isn't a fan of meat, so when he was little I would make sure to balance his diet with lots of plants for ample protein. Once, I went away for a work trip and left my then three-year-old with my mami who came to help. As grandmothers would, she decided she would get him to eat meat. After a couple of tries, she made tiny ground-beef meatballs, adding a little spinach and freshly grated Parmesan cheese, since he loved them both so much, and it worked. At seventeen, he still doesn't love meat, but he still eats grandma's meatballs because they are that good! I like to cook a big batch and store the extra; they can be added to spaghetti sauce, crumbled on a pizza, added to a split hero roll for a quick sandwich, or eaten as is for a snack. They also freeze well. Beyond the taste and flexibility, they also have health benefits, with healing ingredients, such as onions, garlic, and parsley, for antioxidants and vitamins, and added fiber from the spinach.

Preheat the oven to 400°F, with a rack in the middle position.

In a large bowl, beat the egg, then add the ground beef, onion, garlic, Parmesan cheese, bread crumbs, parsley, spinach, Italian seasoning, salt, pepper, milk, and olive oil and mix gently with your hands just until combined.

Shape into about 20 meatballs, about ¼ cup each, or smaller for the little ones, and place on a sheet pan. Bake until just cooked through and lightly browned, 25 to 30 minutes.

NOTE: When making things like meatballs or meatloaf where you can't taste the raw mixture to check the seasonings, here's a workaround: Take a small amount of the mixture and cook it in a small skillet. Taste it and adjust the seasonings as needed.

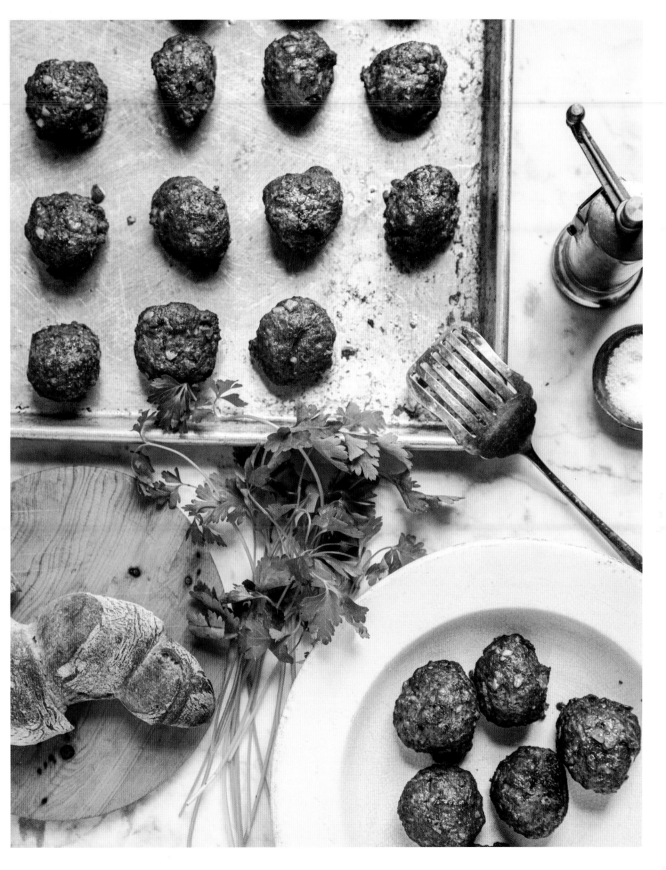

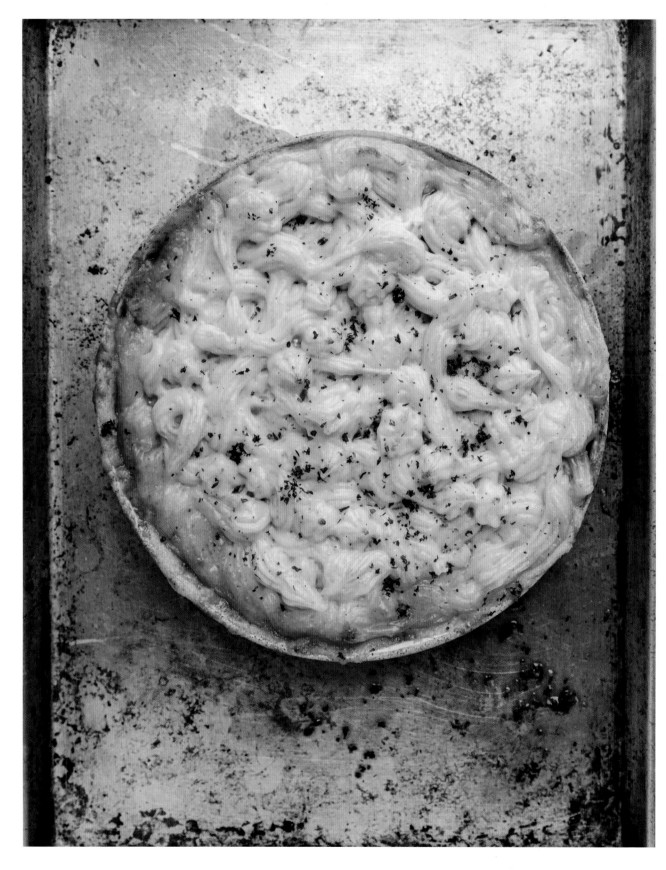

Shepherd's Pie

One of my oldest friends, Clarah, lives in England, and the first time I tried shepherd's pie while visiting her, I fell deeply in love with it, especially the creamy, buttery taste of the mashed-potato topping. The dish is a special treat in our home now. We make it a few times a year and go all out—everything is prepared from scratch following a classic recipe, which includes the healing herbs thyme and rosemary. The only change I made is to substitute Cashew Milk (page 273) for the cream in the potatoes, but they are still dreamy.

Preheat the oven to 400°F.

For the potatoes, place them in a medium pot, cover with about an inch of cold water, and generously season the water with salt. Bring to a boil over high heat, reduce to a simmer, and cook until fork-tender, about 20 minutes. Drain then return the potatoes to the hot pot and let them rest for about 1 minute to allow any remaining liquid to evaporate.

Add the butter, cashew milk, garlic powder, ½ teaspoon of salt, and the pepper and mash until smooth and creamy. Set aside.

For the filling, heat the oil in a large skillet over medium-high heat for 2 minutes. Add the onion and cook, stirring occasionally, until fragrant and translucent, about 5 minutes. Add the meat and break it apart with a wooden spoon. Then add the parsley, rosemary, thyme, salt, and pepper and cook, stirring occasionally, until the meat is no longer pink, 6 to 8 minutes.

Stir in the Worcestershire sauce and garlic and cook for 1 minute. Stir in the flour and tomato paste, making sure there are no lumps, then add the broth and vegetables, cover, and simmer, stirring occasionally, for 5 minutes. Set aside.

To assemble the pie, spread the filling in a large (9 × 13–inch or 7 × 13–inch) baking dish in an even layer. Carefully spoon or pipe the mashed potatoes on top in an even layer. Use a fork to create peaks on the surface, if you like. Bake until browned and bubbling, about 30 minutes. Finish with 1 to 2 minutes under the broiler to further brown those peaks, if you like. Let cool for at least 20 minutes before serving.

MASHED POTATOES

2 pounds russet potatoes (about 2 large), peeled and cut into 1-inch cubes
Sea salt
8 tablespoons (1 stick) butter
⅓ cup Cashew Milk (page 273)
½ teaspoon garlic powder
¼ teaspoon freshly ground black pepper

MEAT FILLING

2 tablespoons olive oil
1 large onion, chopped
2 pounds ground lamb or beef
1 tablespoon chopped fresh flat-leaf parsley
1 teaspoon chopped fresh rosemary leaves
1 teaspoon chopped fresh thyme leaves
½ teaspoon sea salt
½ teaspoon freshly ground black pepper
1 tablespoon Worcestershire sauce
2 cloves garlic, minced
2 tablespoons all-purpose flour
2 tablespoons tomato paste
1 cup low-sodium beef broth
1 cup green beans, cut in ½-inch pieces
1 cup diced (about ¼ inch) carrots
½ cup frozen corn kernels

Beef Bourguignon

This is one dish I truly hope everyone who eats meat will try. The first time I had beef bourguignon was at a café in Paris about twenty-five years ago. My friend and I had walked from the Champs-Élysées and stopped at the first place where we could find a seat. I vividly remember using the crusty bread to soak up the thick sauce, and the succulent beef melting in my mouth. For my girlfriend's Aunty Sherri's fortieth birthday, I made this recipe, which is both comforting and nutrient-dense, and every one of the forty guests asked for my business card, thinking I was a French caterer. Serve with crusty bread or egg noodles.

About 2 hours before cooking, generously season the beef with salt and pepper and let rest until it's almost at room temperature.

Preheat the oven to 350°F.

Heat 2 tablespoons of the butter in a large Dutch oven over medium-high heat. Add the bacon and cook, stirring occasionally, until fully cooked and lightly crisp, 6 to 8 minutes. Transfer the bacon to a plate using a slotted spoon, leaving the drippings in the Dutch oven.

Reheat the drippings over medium heat, if cold, and sear the beef, in batches, as needed, until browned on all sides, 3 to 5 minutes. Be careful not to overcrowd the pot or overlap any pieces or they won't brown properly. Transfer to the plate with the bacon and set aside.

Add 2 tablespoons of the butter and melt over medium heat. Add the carrots, scallions, onions, bay leaves, thyme, 1 teaspoon of salt, and 2 teaspoons of pepper and cook, stirring occasionally, until the onions are lightly browned, 10 to 15 minutes. Add the garlic and cook for 1 minute, stirring.

Add the brandy, step back, and carefully light with a match to burn off the alcohol or avoid this step and allow to slowly reduce as you cook. Add the reserved bacon, beef, and any drippings on the plate. Add the tomato paste and sprinkle in the flour. Stir all the ingredients until no flour is visible.

3 pounds stewing beef, cut into 1-inch cubes and patted dry
Sea salt
Freshly ground black pepper
6 tablespoons (¾ stick) unsalted butter, at room temperature, divided
6 thick slices bacon, diced
5 carrots, cut in thick chunks
4 scallions, chopped
2 onions, chopped
3 bay leaves
1 teaspoon fresh thyme leaves
3 cloves garlic, minced
½ cup brandy
2 tablespoons tomato paste
¼ cup all-purpose flour
2 cups good dry red wine, such as a Côtes du Rhône or Pinot Noir
2 cups low-sodium beef broth
1 pound cremini mushrooms, sliced
1 pound frozen pearl onions

(Continued)

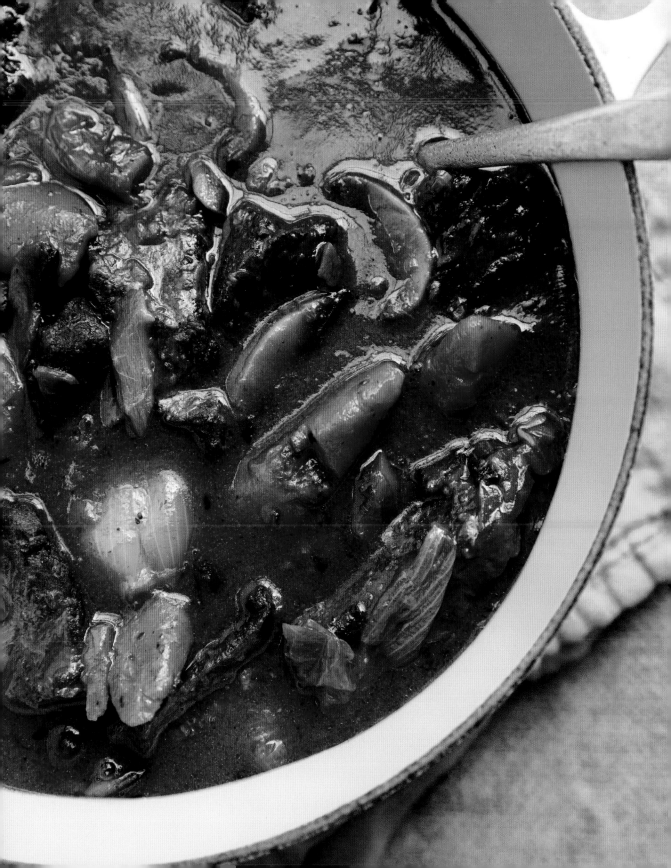

Add the wine and beef broth to barely cover the meat. Bring to a simmer, cover the pot with a tight-fitting lid, and bake until the meat and vegetables are very tender when pierced with a fork, about 1¼ hours.

Meanwhile, melt the remaining 2 tablespoons of butter in a large skillet over medium heat. Add the mushrooms, season to taste with salt and pepper, and cook, stirring occasionally, until the mushrooms are tender and lightly browned, about 10 minutes.

Stir the mushrooms and pearl onions into the beef bourguignon, season to taste, and bake until thick and bubbly, about 30 minutes more. Adjust the seasonings, if needed, and let sit for 15 minutes before serving.

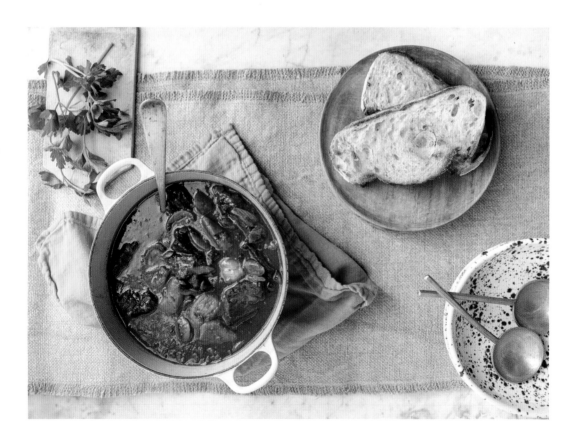

Sheet Pan Flank Steak with Carrots and Potatoes

4 small carrots, peeled, cut into 1½-inch chunks on the bias

4 small unpeeled red potatoes, quartered

3 tablespoons olive oil, divided

Sea salt

Freshly ground black pepper

Crushed red pepper flakes (optional)

1 pound flank steak

2 teaspoons chopped fresh thyme leaves

I love a great sheet pan recipe for the ease it affords me to make either a quick side of Kale Salad (page 249) or Quinoa with Cilantro and Lemon (page 242) while the bulk of my dinner cooks. Flank steak is one of the healthiest beef cuts—ounce for ounce it has fewer calories and more protein than a rib eye, according to my local butcher. What I know for sure is that it is super flavorful, chock-full of protein, vitamins, and minerals, including B_6, B_{12}, selenium, iron, and zinc. The carrots and potatoes add fiber and other nutrients to this dish. This can be a meal, though at our home we love to stretch it to save a little for leftovers by serving it with a salad, quinoa, or Stir-Fried Cauliflower Rice (page 241).

Preheat the broiler, with a rack about 6 inches from the heat.

In a large bowl, toss together the carrots, potatoes, 1 tablespoon of the oil, salt and black pepper to taste, and red pepper flakes, if using. Spread in an even layer across a sheet pan, then place a wire rack over the veggies.

Rub the steak with the remaining 2 tablespoons of oil, thyme, 1 teaspoon of salt, and ½ teaspoon of pepper, or to taste. Broil for 10 minutes, then flip the steak, Broil until desired doneness, about 5 minutes more for medium-rare.

Transfer the steak to a cutting board and let rest for about 5 minutes while the potatoes and carrots finish cooking, if necessary. Cut the steak across the grain into thin slices and place in a large serving bowl. Stir the vegetables in the delicious juices in the sheet pan, then transfer the vegetables and the juices to the bowl with the meat, gently toss together, and serve.

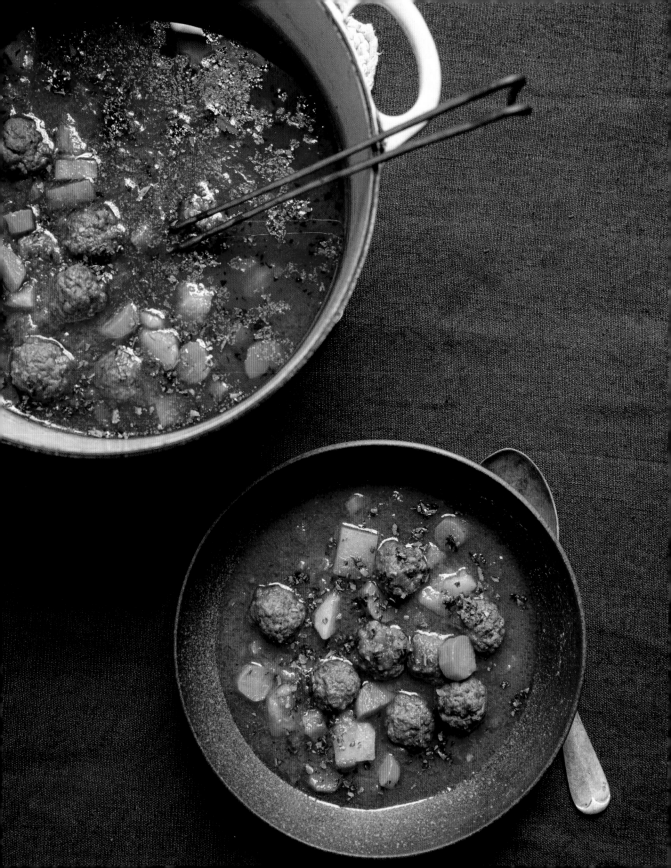

GF, DF

SERVES 6 TO 8

1 pound ground beef
1 onion
1½ teaspoons sea salt,
   divided
½ teaspoon garlic
   powder
2 tablespoons olive oil
1 teaspoon ground
   turmeric
3 tablespoons tomato
   paste
4 cups low-sodium
   chicken broth
3 cups chopped
   tomatoes or
   1 (28-ounce) can
   diced tomatoes
2 or 3 medium carrots
   (about ½ pound),
   peeled and cut into
   1-inch cubes
½ pound russet
   potatoes, peeled and
   cut into 1-inch cubes
¼ cup chopped fresh
   flat-leaf parsley

Kalleh Gonjeeshki

PERSIAN MEATBALL AND POTATO SOUP

This is a simple, comforting Iranian dish of beef meatballs and potatoes simmered in a tomato sauce. "Kalleh gonjeeshki" means "sparrow's head" in Persian, and here references the size of the meatballs. Every family has its own version of this favorite. This version is from my beautiful Iranian friend Ghazaleh. It hits the spot every time, and I love that it is chock-full of nutrients, including a scientifically proven anti-inflammatory compound from turmeric. Serve with crusty bread or rice.

Break the ground beef into small pieces into a large bowl and set aside.

Cut the onion in half. Dice half of the onion and transfer to a small bowl. Cut the remaining half of the onion into 2 wedges. Dice 1 onion wedge and add it to the diced onions. Grate the remaining onion wedge, using the large holes of a box grater, and add it to the ground beef.

Sprinkle 1 teaspoon of the salt and the garlic powder over the ground beef and onions. Mix with your hands until fully combined and set aside.

Heat the olive oil in a large Dutch oven over medium heat. Add the diced onions and the remaining ½ teaspoon of salt and cook, stirring occasionally, until translucent and starting to brown, 3 to 5 minutes. If the bottom of the pot starts to turn dark, deglaze with a little water.

Add the turmeric and cook, stirring occasionally, until fragrant, about 30 seconds. Add the tomato paste and cook, stirring often, until the paste turns dark red, 3 to 5 minutes. Add the chicken broth and tomatoes and break up the tomatoes a bit with a wooden spoon. Bring the liquid to a simmer over medium-high heat.

Meanwhile, roll the beef mixture into small meatballs, using about 1 to 2 teaspoons of meat per ball. Gently place the meatballs into the broth, cover, and simmer for 20 minutes over low heat.

Add the carrots and potatoes to the broth and simmer, uncovered, until the vegetables are tender, 20 to 30 minutes more. Check the seasonings and garnish with the parsley. Serve.

MAINS | MEAT   149

4 cloves garlic, minced
3½ teaspoons finely
    chopped fresh
    rosemary leaves
3½ teaspoons finely
    chopped fresh
    thyme leaves
2½ teaspoons sea salt
2 tablespoons
    unsalted butter,
    melted
1 tablespoon olive oil
1½ to 2½ pounds rack
    of lamb (8 to 10 ribs),
    frenched

Skillet–Roasted Rack of Lamb with Herbs

If I had to pick one meat dish to eat for the rest of my life, it would be this rack of lamb, which is coated with herbs, garlic, and melted butter, then seared and roasted to juicy, tender perfection. The simplicity reminds me of a famous quote from Julia Child: "You don't have to cook fancy or complicated masterpieces, just good food from fresh ingredients." The dish is high in anti-inflammatory properties thanks to the rosemary and thyme, as well as the omega-3 and zinc from the lamb. Serve with Herbed Parmesan French Fries (page 258) and Turmeric Garlicky Mayo (page 259). You can also enjoy the lamb with any of my salads or Stir-Fried Cauliflower Rice (page 241), depending on what you are in the mood for.

In a small bowl, stir together the garlic, herbs, salt, and butter. Rub the mixture all over the lamb, then refrigerate, covered, for at least 2 hours or up to 1 day.

Take the lamb out of the fridge about 20 minutes before you plan to cook it and preheat the oven to 400°F.

Meanwhile, grease the bottom of a large skillet with the oil and place the skillet over medium-high heat. Add the lamb and sear for 1 to 2 minutes on each side, depending on the size. Move the skillet into the oven and roast for 14 to 16 minutes for medium-rare, 145°F on a meat thermometer (or less or more, as desired). Transfer the rack to a platter, cover, and let rest for about 5 minutes before serving.

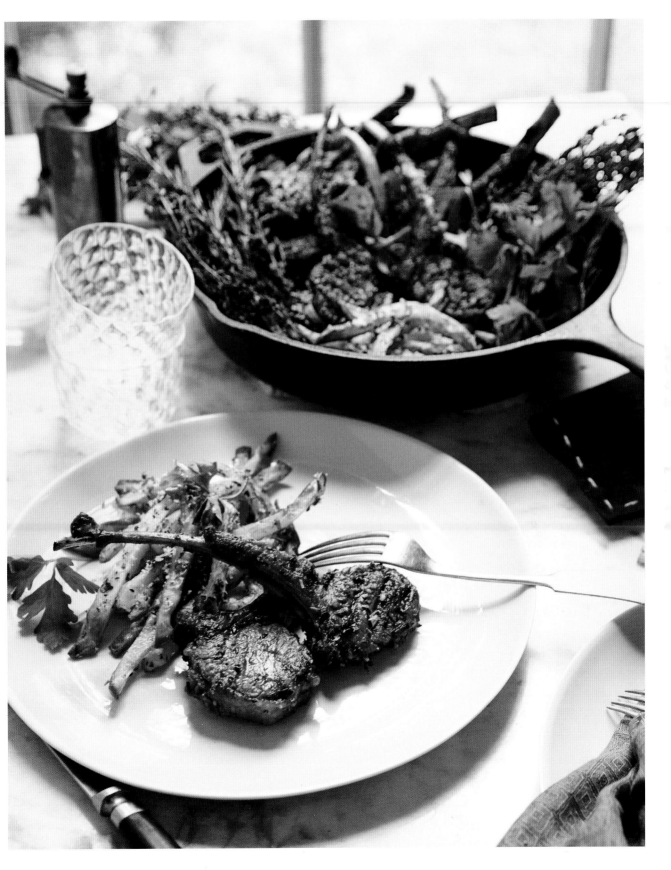

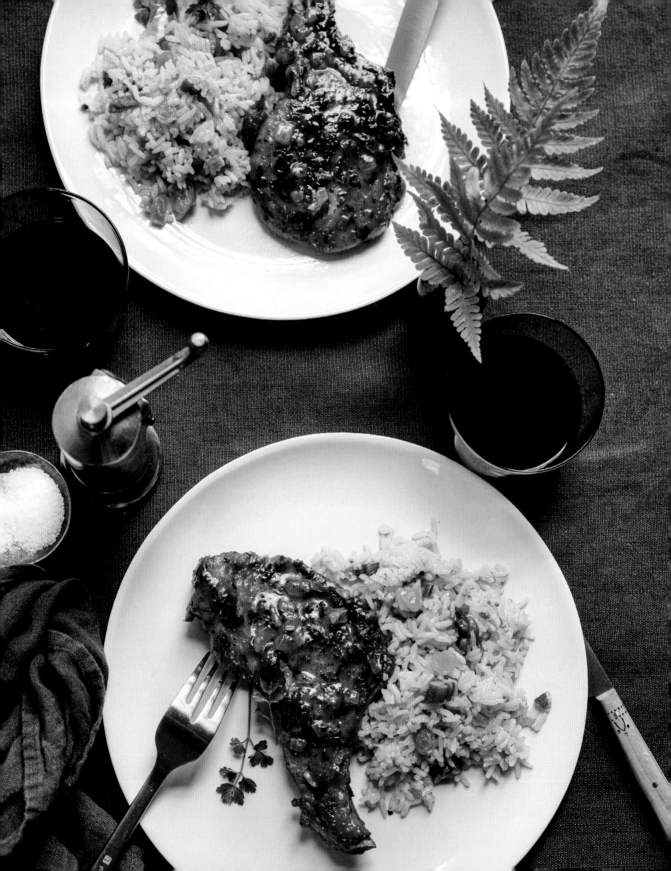

4 (5- to 6-ounce) bone-in, center-cut pork chops, about ½ inch thick
1 teaspoon sea salt
½ teaspoon freshly ground black pepper
¼ cup all-purpose flour
4 teaspoons olive oil, divided
1 onion, chopped
3 cloves garlic, minced
2 cups low-sodium chicken or beef broth
1 tablespoon finely chopped fresh flat-leaf parsley
1 tablespoon chopped fresh rosemary leaves
1 tablespoon chopped fresh thyme leaves

Braised Pork Chops and Herbs

These tender juicy braised pork chops, seasoned with fresh herbs, make a perfect dish that can be paired with any of my sides. No matter what you pair them with, the taste is amazing for such an easy dish to pull together. Besides being high in protein, pork is also rich in essential vitamins and minerals. I recommend using pasture-raised pork, for both nutrition and taste. The difference between that and factory-raised pork is like night and day. In fact, the first time I tasted the latter after moving to the States, I didn't even realize it was pork! Pasture-raised pork is pricier, but if given the choice, I'd rather have less of the good stuff. Serve the chops with Nutty Spiced Rice (page 245), Stir-Fried Cauliflower Rice (page 241), or Plantain Tapé (page 255).

Sprinkle the pork chops with the salt and pepper. Dust with the flour, shake off any excess, and set aside.

In a large skillet, heat 2 teaspoons of oil over medium heat. Add the pork chops and cook until browned, about 4 minutes per side, flipping once. Transfer to a plate and set aside, reserving the skillet.

In the same skillet, heat the remaining 2 teaspoons of oil over medium heat. Add the onion and cook, stirring occasionally, just until translucent, about 4 minutes. Add the garlic and cook, stirring, for about 30 seconds more.

Add the broth and herbs and scrape up any crusty bits on the bottom of the pan with a wooden spatula. Add the pork chops, reduce the heat, and gently simmer until just cooked through, registering 135°F on a meat thermometer (if you have time for it to rest for 10 minutes) and 147°F if the family is waiting, 10 to 15 minutes.

Serve.

Lamb Lasagna with Spinach and Feta

This Greek-inspired recipe, a family favorite, ticks all the boxes: It is easy, delicious, belly warming, and nourishing, it can be made ahead of time, and it reheats well. Try to use grass-fed lamb, if possible. It's one of the richest sources of an essential fatty acid that helps improve immune-system health and contains a greater amount of omega-3 fats than factory-farm lamb. Not only do omega-3 fats play a crucial role in bone health and joint health by boosting the amount of calcium in your bones, but they also help control rheumatoid arthritis symptoms and decrease the risk of heart disease. Feel free to leave out the spinach if you can't have it, but I would encourage you to give it a try. It adds color, taste, and nutrients to this dish.

Preheat the oven to 375°F.

In a large skillet, heat the oil over medium heat. Add the onions and cook, stirring occasionally, until translucent, about 5 minutes. Add the garlic and cook, stirring, for about 30 seconds. Add the lamb and rosemary and cook, breaking up the meat with a wooden spoon and stirring occasionally, until the meat is browned, about 14 minutes more.

Stir in the broth and simmer, scraping the bottom of the pan to remove any crusty bits, until slightly reduced, about 3 minutes. Stir in the tomatoes, salt, and pepper and bring to a boil over high heat, then reduce the heat and simmer the sauce until the seasoning combines, about 4 minutes more. Taste and adjust the seasoning as needed.

Meanwhile, in a small bowl, stir together the ricotta and lemon zest. Spread the top of each lasagna noodle with about 2 tablespoons of the ricotta mixture.

Lightly coat an 11 × 7–inch glass or ceramic baking dish with oil, then evenly cover the bottom with 2 cups of the sauce.

Ingredients

- 2 teaspoons olive oil, plus more for greasing the baking dish
- 1½ cups chopped onions
- 3 cloves garlic, minced
- 1 pound ground lamb
- 1 tablespoon chopped fresh rosemary leaves
- 1¼ cups low-sodium chicken broth
- 2½ pounds tomatoes, chopped, or 3 (14-ounce) cans crushed tomatoes
- ¾ teaspoon sea salt
- ½ teaspoon freshly ground black pepper
- 1¼ cups ricotta cheese
- ½ teaspoon grated lemon zest
- 9 no-boil lasagna noodles
- 2 cups finely chopped spinach
- ¾ cup crumbled feta cheese
- ¼ cup fresh flat-leaf parsley

Arrange 3 lasagna noodles, ricotta-side up, over the sauce, then top with 2 more cups of the sauce and half of the spinach. Repeat twice. Then add a final layer of sauce.

Sprinkle the top of the lasagna with feta cheese, cover with parchment paper and foil, and bake until bubbly and the noodles are tender, about 40 minutes. Remove the cover and let stand for about 10 minutes before sprinkling with the parsley, cutting, and serving.

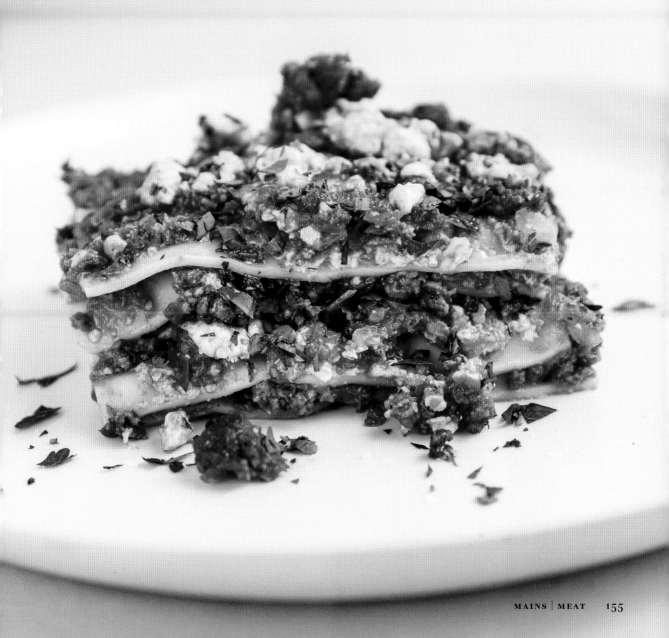

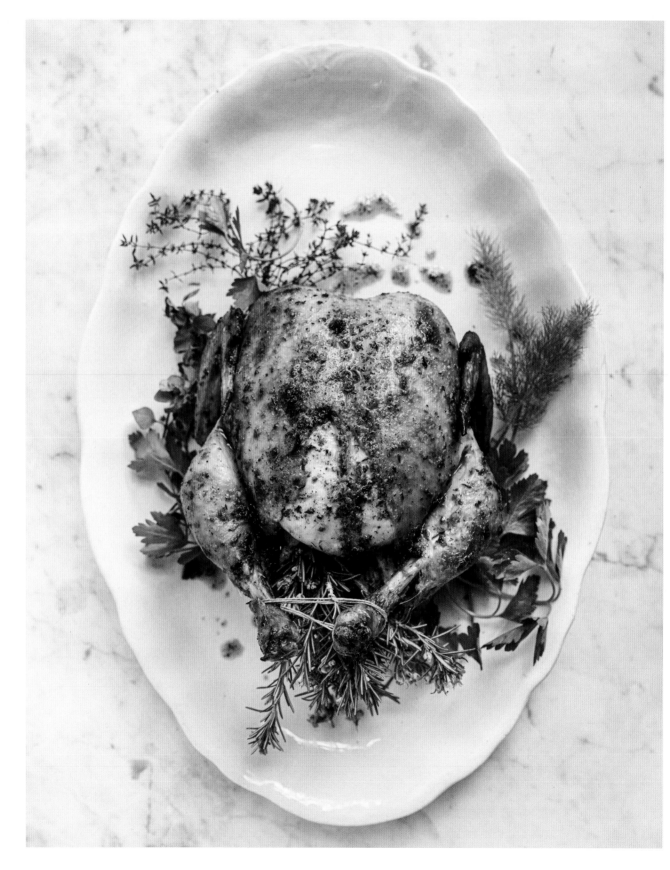

Roasted Chicken

Roasting a whole chicken makes meal planning for the week super easy even if you live alone. If you buy rotisserie chicken, this recipe is a healthier option since your chicken doesn't get soaked in the brining solution, which often has added sugar. Even when a recipe calls for a specific part of the chicken, I always buy a whole chicken and butcher it myself at home. It's simple to do, is usually much more economical, and you get all the bones, which can be used to make stock. Before I moved to the States, I didn't even know you could buy cut-up chicken! Use any leftover meat in tacos, salads, sandwiches, or whatever else you can think of. It's also great in my Chicken Pot Pie (page 168). And even though the bones have been roasted, you can still make broth with them.

If you can afford it, please consider buying pasture-raised chicken. The meat contains 50 percent more vitamin A, which supports your immune system, and about 30 percent less saturated fat than conventionally raised chicken, and the taste and texture are so much better. Enjoy this with Stir-Fried Cauliflower Rice (page 241) or with any of the salads.

2 tablespoons olive oil, plus more for greasing the pan
4 cloves garlic, minced
1 tablespoon finely chopped fresh rosemary leaves
1 tablespoon finely chopped fresh thyme leaves
1 teaspoon onion powder
1 teaspoon Bragg Liquid Aminos
1½ teaspoons sea salt
1 teaspoon freshly ground black pepper
1 (3½- to 4-pound) whole chicken, at room temperature, patted dry and giblet bag (if there is one) removed
5 sprigs rosemary
1 lemon, halved

Preheat the oven to 425°F, with a rack in the middle position. Lightly grease a roasting rack with olive oil set in a roasting pan. (If you don't have a rack, that's fine. Lightly grease the bottom of the pan. The bottom of the bird won't brown as well that way, but you can always broil it for a few minutes, if you like.)

In a small bowl, stir together the oil, garlic, chopped rosemary, thyme, onion powder, aminos, salt, and pepper. Rub the mixture all over the chicken, under the skin (gently separate the skin from the meat with your fingertips), and in the cavity. Place the rosemary sprigs and the lemon halves in the cavity, then tie the legs together with butcher's twine (optional).

Place the chicken breast-side up in the prepared pan and roast until the juices run clear and the meat is just cooked through, until the thickest part reaches 165°F on a meat thermometer, about 1 hour 15 minutes, turning the chicken halfway through and basting every 15 minutes.

Let rest for about 20 minutes before carving.

One-Skillet, Date-Night Lemony Chicken

1 tablespoon olive oil
4 bone-in, skin-on chicken thighs or 2 breasts, at room temperature and patted dry
1 teaspoon sea salt
½ teaspoon freshly ground black pepper
4 unpeeled Yukon gold potatoes (about 1 pound), halved
1 bunch broccolini (about 10 ounces)
4 cloves garlic
2 lemons, sliced and seeded
2 sprigs rosemary
1 cup dry white wine
2 tablespoons unsalted butter, cut into pieces

After Georges and I had kids and it became more challenging to go out, I started looking for creative ways to make our date nights at home feel more like an actual event. Preparing a special meal just for us was an easy solution, as long as it was delicious, but not too involved—after all, we were still tired and on borrowed time most nights! This recipe, which only calls for basic ingredients and one pan, quickly became a favorite for both of us. I hope you like it as much as we do. (We also share some with the kids when we are feeling generous.) Potatoes are left unpeeled for added nutrients. You won't want to let a drop of the light, buttery lemony sauce go to waste; the hint of butter makes it so dreamy.

Preheat the oven to 400°F, with a rack in the middle position.

In a large cast-iron skillet, heat the oil over medium-high heat until very hot.

Sprinkle the chicken with the salt and pepper, place it skin-side down in the skillet, and cook until the skin is golden brown, 5 to 7 minutes. Flip the chicken and cook until browned, about 5 minutes.

Off the heat, arrange the potatoes, broccolini, garlic, lemon slices, and rosemary sprigs around the chicken. Using a pot holder wiggle the skillet a little to mix and settle the potatoes, and bake until the chicken is just cooked through, 165°F on a meat thermometer, and the potatoes are tender, about 40 minutes.

Place a pot holder over the handle of the skillet for the next steps because it will be very hot. Divide the chicken, vegetables, and lemon slices between two plates. Discard the rosemary. Heat the skillet over medium-high heat and cook the pan juices until almost evaporated. Add the wine and deglaze the skillet, scraping the bottom with a spoon to get up any crusty bits and crush the garlic. Simmer the wine until it is reduced by about half. Add the butter and whisk. Turn off the heat. Adjust the seasonings if necessary and pour the sauce over the chicken and vegetables. Serve.

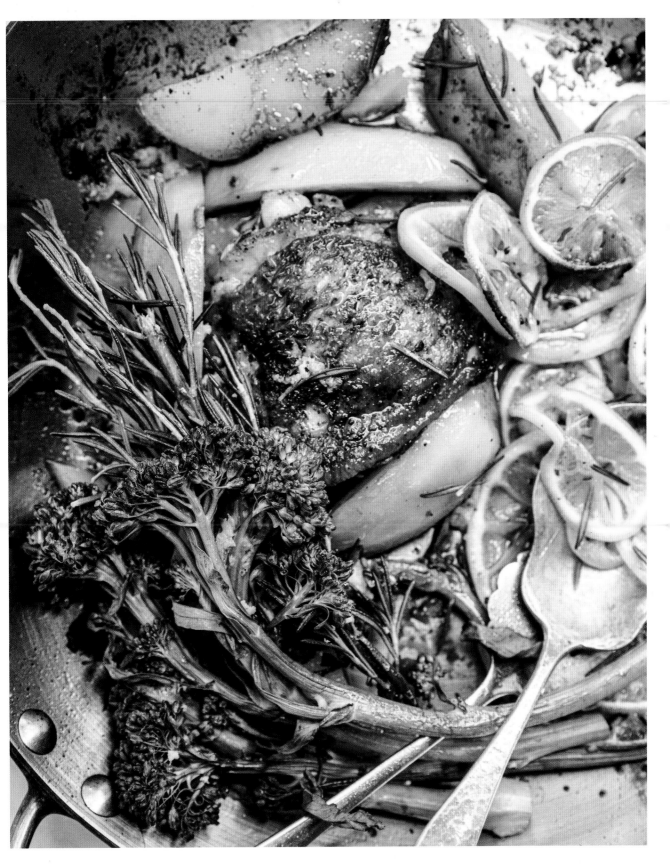

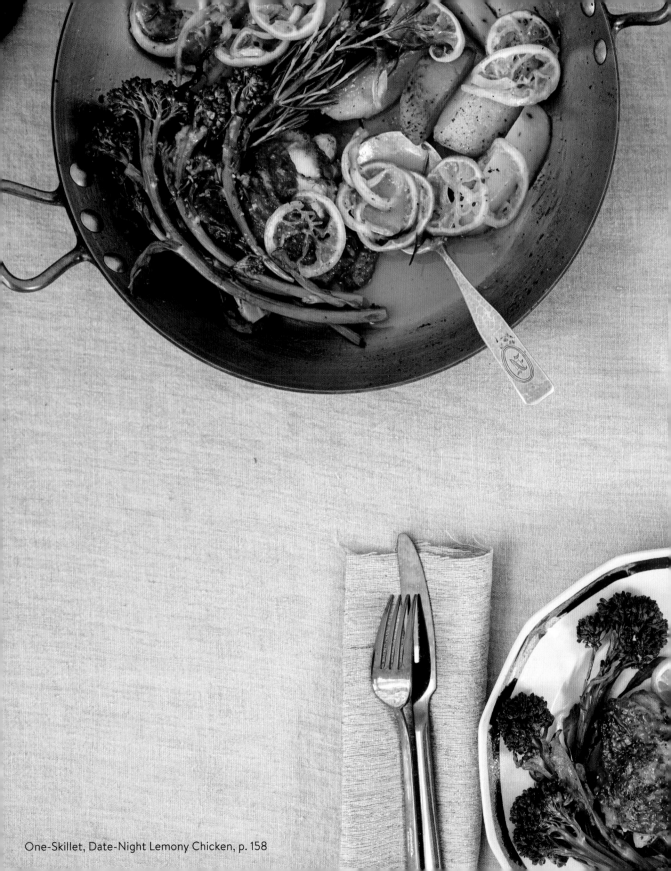

One-Skillet, Date-Night Lemony Chicken, p. 158

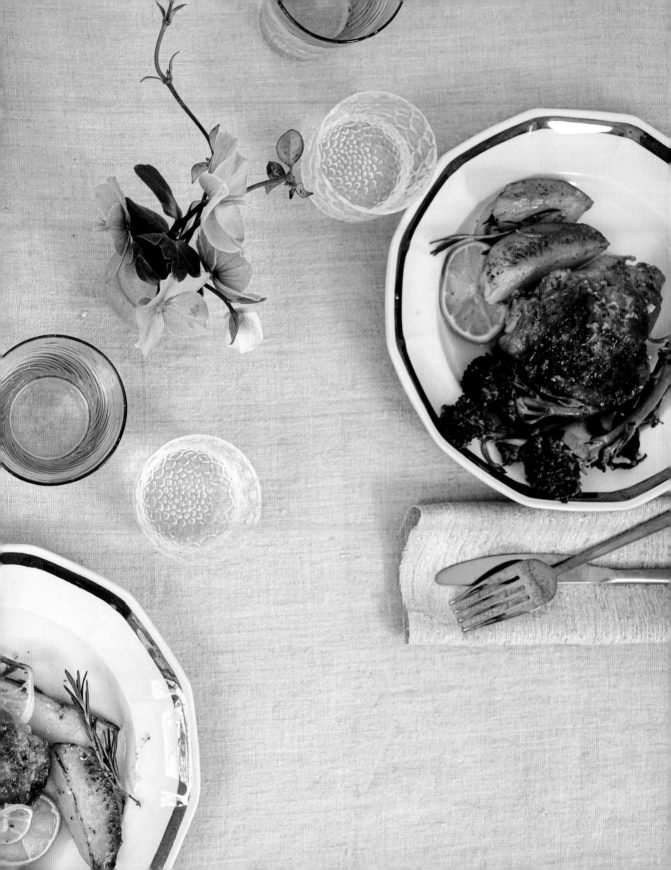

Okra Stew

Okra is a flowering plant that is completely edible and very popular in Africa and here in the southern states. Did you know okra is an indigenous West African vegetable that has spread globally? The English word "okra" is derived from the Twi word "nkuruma." Okra is famous in the United Stated as the thickening agent in the gumbo stews of Louisiana. The French word for okra is "gombo," which, like gumbo itself, derives from a Bantu word. I grew up eating okra in so many different ways, but my favorite to this day is this mouthwatering, thick, tomato-based stew my mami made with either fresh fish or chicken. The secret to this dish was the fresh cutmanjo (basil) she would have us harvest from the garden. Okra stew to me is soul food at its finest, packed with nutrients and incredible taste, and so economical. If you are still on the fence about okra, I ask that you give this recipe a try. Make it with beef, fish, chicken, or oyster mushrooms. If you love the Louisiana gumbo you are going to love this dish even more. While you can absolutely use frozen okra, I highly recommend fresh; the taste is so refreshingly good. Enjoy with Stir-Fried Cauliflower Rice (page 241), Quinoa with Cilantro and Lemon (page 242), Nutty Spiced Rice (page 245), or whatever you like.

In a medium pot, combine the chicken, half the onions, half the garlic, 1 teaspoon of salt, or to taste, ginger, thyme, rosemary, and water. Cover and cook on medium-high heat until chicken is cooked, about 10 minutes, and set side.

In a medium skillet, heat the oil over medium heat, add the remaining onions and leeks and cook, stirring occasionally, until translucent, about 5 minutes. Add the remaining garlic and cook, stirring, for about 1 minute. Add the tomatoes and continue cooking for about 10 minutes, stirring as needed to avoid sticking to the bottom of the pan.

Remove the thyme and rosemary stems from the chicken and discard them. Pour everything from the pot into the skillet, add the red pepper flakes, if using, Better Than Bouillon, smoked paprika, and black pepper

2 chicken breasts (about 1 pound), cut into 1-inch cubes
2 onions, diced, divided
4 cloves garlic, minced, divided
Sea salt
1-inch piece fresh ginger, grated (about 1 teaspoon)
5 sprigs thyme
1 sprig rosemary
2 cups water
⅓ cup olive oil
⅓ cup chopped leeks
1 pound tomatoes, diced (about 6 tomatoes)
½ teaspoon crushed red pepper flakes or 1 small habanero (optional)
1 teaspoon Better Than Bouillon or coconut aminos
½ pound okra (about 8 spears) tough stems removed and cut into 3 or 4 pieces, depending on length
2 scallions, diced
1 cup low-sodium chicken broth
⅓ cup chopped fresh basil
1 teaspoon smoked paprika
Freshly ground black pepper

and bring to a boil. Add the okra, scallions, and broth and stir. Cover and allow to simmer for 5 minutes. Add the basil, stir, and cook for 1 minute more. Adjust the seasoning to taste and serve. While we prefer our okra crisp-tender, please feel free to cook longer if you like yours more tender.

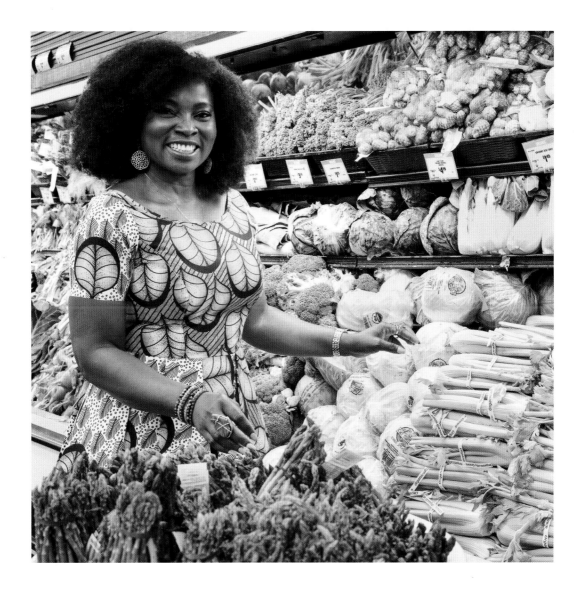

Poulet DG

DIRECTOR GENERAL'S CHICKEN

Chicken braised with colorful vegetables, herbs, and fried plantains was one of my favorite dishes when I was growing up in Cameroon and it still is to this day. Because of the breadth and amount of ingredients it required, the dish was only served on special occasions, hence its name. The only changes I made to this incredible dish to fit my current lifestyle without compromising the taste is baking or air frying the chicken and plantains instead of frying them in oil. I also replaced the traditional Maggi seasoning with Bragg Liquid Aminos. Other than that, this dish was already bursting with all types of amazing nutrients. (If you have an air fryer, you can cook the chicken and plantains in there, separately.)

Preheat the oven to 400°F. Line a sheet pan with parchment paper.

For the chicken, combine all the ingredients in a large pot and toss together. Bring to a boil over high heat, then reduce the heat to medium, cover, and steam for 15 to 20 minutes, stirring occasionally to avoid sticking to the bottom. Transfer the chicken to the prepared sheet pan in a single layer using tongs and reserve the broth. Bake the chicken until lightly browned, 15 to 20 minutes.

Meanwhile, line another sheet pan with parchment and toss the plantains with oil and salt on the prepared pan in a single layer. Bake at 400°F until tender and golden, 30 to 35 minutes, flipping halfway.

While the chicken and plantains cook, prepare the tomato base. Heat the oil in a large skillet over medium-high heat. Add the leek and onion and sauté, stirring occasionally, until fragrant, about 7 minutes. Add the garlic and cook, stirring occasionally, for 1 minute more.

CHICKEN

- 1 (4-pound) chicken, cut into medium-sized pieces (16 to 20 pieces)
- 2 cloves garlic, minced
- 1 large onion, diced
- 1 tablespoon chopped fresh rosemary leaves
- 1 tablespoon chopped fresh thyme leaves
- 1 teaspoon Bragg Liquid Aminos
- 1 teaspoon grated peeled fresh ginger
- 1½ teaspoons sea salt

PLANTAINS

- 4 semi-ripe plantains, peeled and diced
- 1 tablespoon olive oil
- ½ teaspoon sea salt

TOMATO BASE

- ¼ cup olive oil
- 1 small leek, pale green and white parts thinly sliced
- 1 large onion, diced
- 2 cloves garlic, minced
- 1 pound Roma tomatoes, diced
- 1 or 2 Scotch bonnet peppers (optional)
- 8 ounces green beans, cut into 2-inch pieces
- 3 carrots, quartered and cut into 2-inch pieces
- 1 red bell pepper, seeded and sliced
- 1 yellow bell pepper, seeded and sliced
- 1 teaspoon Bragg Liquid Aminos
- ½ teaspoon sea salt
- 2 to 4 tablespoons low-sodium chicken broth, if needed

Add the tomatoes and Scotch bonnet, if using, and cook, stirring occasionally, until the liquid is almost gone, about 10 minutes. (Mash the Scotch bonnet with a spoon to break it into tiny pieces.) Add the green beans and carrots and cook, stirring occasionally, until almost tender, about 4 minutes. Add the browned chicken, reserved broth, plantains, bell peppers, aminos, and salt and stir to combine. Cook for 3 minutes more. Taste and adjust the seasonings. Add a little chicken broth if the dish is too dry, for that moist texture this dish is known for. Serve.

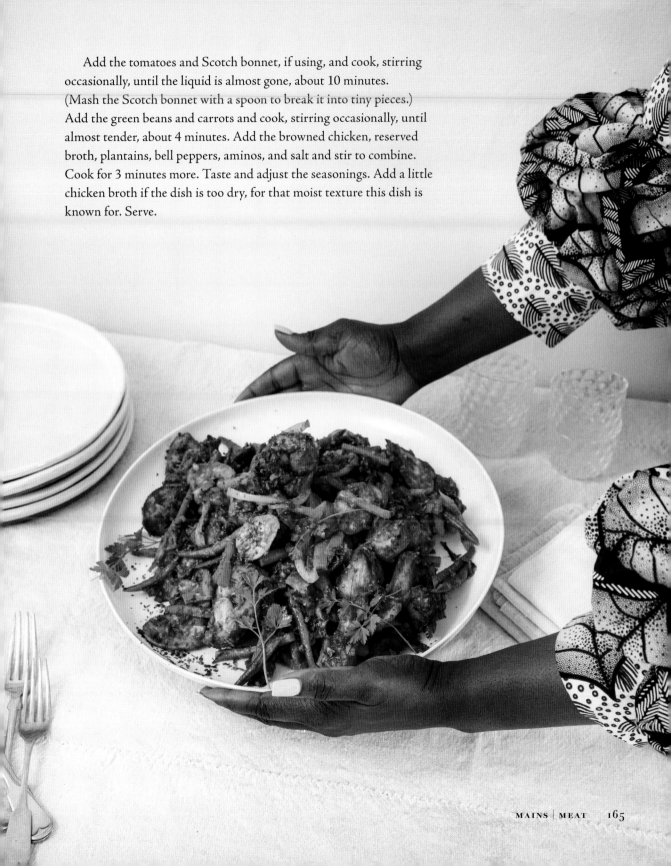

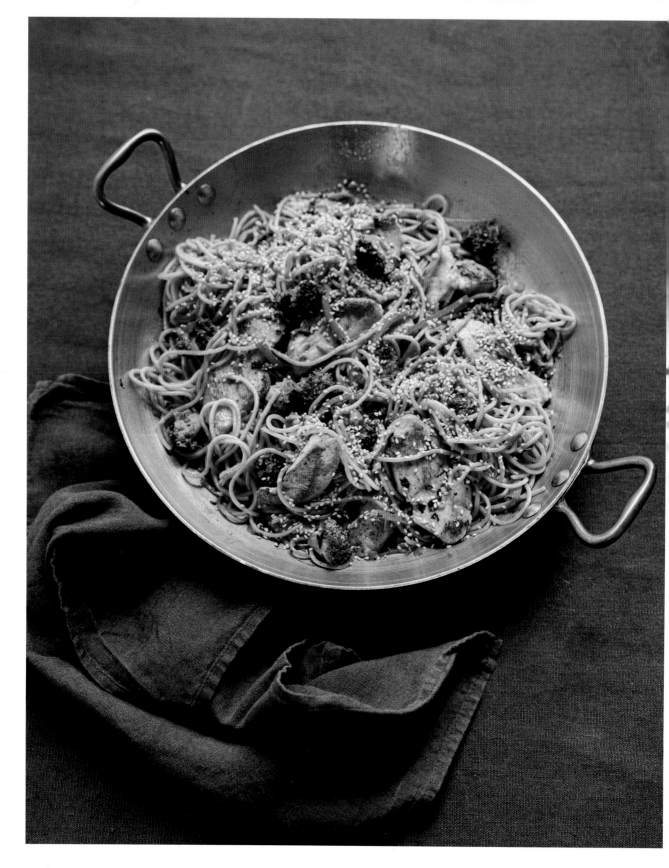

Chicken, Vegetable, and Noodle Stir-Fry

Children, including my own, generally love noodles. Often, they'll even eat them if you toss them with other ingredients they might not like on their own, such as vegetables. As such, I've had good success serving this Asian-style veggie-packed dish to picky eaters. I also keep it as wholesome as possible by using 100 percent whole grain pasta (such as whole wheat, lentil, chickpea, etc.). If you or your kids aren't fans of that, I do encourage you to give it another go in this recipe. There are so many other ingredients and flavors that you may not mind it. And it's worth a try because whole grain pasta provides many important nutritional benefits, including vitamins, antioxidants, fiber, protein, and healthy fats, that white "enriched" pasta is devoid of.

Bring a medium pot of salted water to a boil.

Meanwhile, make the sauce. In a small bowl, stir together all the ingredients and set aside.

For the stir-fry, when the water comes to a boil, cook the spaghetti according to the package directions. When about 3 minutes are left, add the broccoli and stir. Right before draining the pasta and broccoli, stir in the kale, then drain and set aside.

In a medium skillet, heat the oil over medium heat. Season the chicken with salt and pepper, then place it in the skillet in a single layer and cook until slightly golden on both sides, 2 to 3 minutes, turning occasionally.

Add the onion and cook, stirring occasionally, for about 3 minutes, then add the scallions, garlic, and carrot and cook until the chicken is just cooked through, about 1 minute more.

Add the cooked spaghetti, broccoli, and kale and toss, then pour the sauce over the ingredients and gently toss until evenly combined and the spaghetti is heated through, about 2 minutes more. Serve garnished with the sesame seeds.

SAUCE

- ¼ cup tamari
- 2 tablespoons hoisin sauce
- 1 tablespoon maple syrup
- 2 teaspoons toasted sesame oil
- ½ teaspoon grated peeled fresh ginger
- ¼ teaspoon crushed red pepper flakes (optional)
- ¼ teaspoon freshly ground black pepper

STIR-FRY

- ½ pound 100 percent whole grain spaghetti
- 3 cups broccoli florets
- 2 cups chopped baby kale
- 2 tablespoons olive oil
- 1 pound boneless, skinless chicken breasts, cut lengthwise into ¼-inch-wide strips
- Sea salt
- Freshly ground black pepper
- ½ onion, finely chopped
- 4 scallions, thinly sliced
- 3 cloves garlic, minced
- 1 large carrot, julienned
- 1 tablespoon toasted sesame seeds

Chicken Pot Pie

If your family likes chicken pot pie, this recipe is probably a little more wholesome than most. The finished pies are so beautiful, no one will believe how easy they are to make. (You can use the meat from my Roasted Chicken on page 157, or, if you're very busy, you can start with a store-bought rotisserie chicken.) For an equally beautiful and delicious vegetarian version, replace the chicken and chicken broth with oyster mushrooms and veggie broth, respectively.

Start with the dough for the crust. In a small bowl or cup, combine the water and 10 ice cubes and allow the cubes to melt a little to make the water even colder. (This helps create a tender, flaky result.)

Sift the flour and salt into a food processor and pulse 3 to 5 times. Add the butter and pulse until the mixture resembles a coarse meal with some pea-sized pieces of butter.

With the food processor running, add 1 tablespoon of the ice water at a time through the chute until a dough forms (watch the dough closely). Turn the dough out onto a lightly floured surface and knead for just about a minute. Form the dough into a ball, divide it into 4 balls if using individual ramekins, flatten to make rolling easier later, and wrap in plastic wrap. Place in the refrigerator for about 30 minutes.

Preheat the oven to 400°F, with a rack in the center of the oven.

On a sheet pan, toss together the oil, carrots, celery, onions, ½ teaspoon of salt, and ¼ teaspoon of pepper and bake until tender and lightly browned, about 30 minutes.

Meanwhile, lightly grease four 8-ounce ovenproof ramekins with oil, place them on a baking sheet, and set aside.

In a medium pot, melt the butter over low heat, then whisk in the flour and cook, whisking constantly, for 1 minute. Gradually whisk in the broth and gently simmer over medium heat, whisking constantly, until smooth and slightly thickened, about 5 minutes.

CRUST

- ⅓ cup plus 1 tablespoon water
- 10 ice cubes
- 2 cups all-purpose flour, plus more for rolling out the dough
- 1½ teaspoons sea salt
- 12 tablespoons (1½ sticks) cold unsalted butter, cut into small pieces
- 1 large egg beaten with 1 tablespoon water

FILLING

- 3 tablespoons olive oil, plus more for greasing the ramekins
- 1 pound carrots, cut into ½-inch dice
- 5 stalks celery, cut into ½-inch dice
- 2 small onions, diced
- Sea salt
- Freshly ground black pepper
- 8 tablespoons (1 stick) unsalted butter
- ½ cup all-purpose flour
- 4 cups low-sodium chicken broth
- 4 cups shredded cooked white and/or dark chicken meat
- 2 cups frozen peas
- 1½ teaspoons fresh thyme leaves

(Continued)

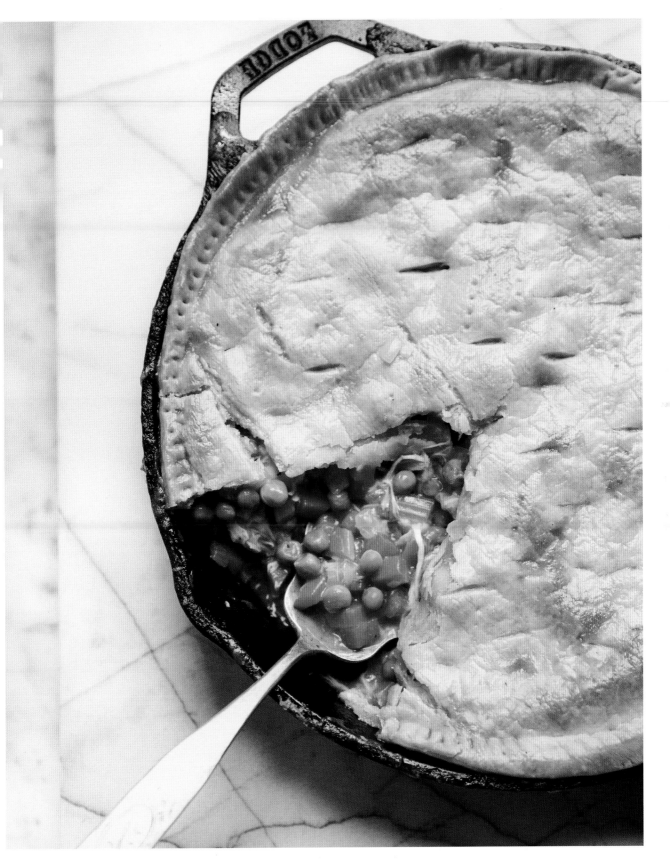

Stir in the roasted vegetables, chicken, peas, thyme, ½ teaspoon of salt, and ¼ teaspoon of pepper and cook, stirring occassionally, until thickened and bubbly, about 10 minutes. Divide the hot filling among the prepared ramekins.

Roll out the pie dough on a lightly floured surface. Lay a crust on top of each filled ramekin and trim the edges as needed. Brush the dough with egg wash and cut a slit in the top. Bake on the baking sheet until the dough is golden brown, about 30 minutes. Let the pot pie cool for a few minutes, then serve.

NOTE: If you do not have four 8-ounce ramekins, you can make one large pot pie in a 10-inch cast-iron skillet or 3-quart baking dish, adjusting the baking time as needed for the dough to become golden brown.

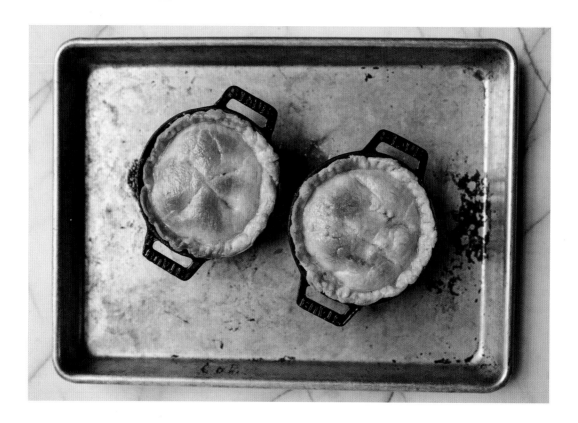

1 tablespoon maple
  syrup
1 teaspoon raw honey
  (see Note)
1 tablespoon Dijon
  mustard
1 tablespoon chopped
  fresh sage, divided
4 bone-in, skin-on split
  chicken breasts
Sea salt
4 unpeeled red
  potatoes (about
  1 pound), cut into
  1-inch dice
2 carrots, peeled and
  cut into 1-inch dice
1 large sweet onion,
  quartered
½ acorn squash,
  seeded and cut
  crosswise into 1-inch
  slices
10 Brussels sprouts
  (about ½ pound),
  quartered
2 tablespoons olive oil
1 teaspoon freshly
  ground black pepper,
  divided

Maple-Glazed Chicken and Veggies

This has to be one of my all-time favorite recipes to cook, not because it is high in protein from the chicken and fiber and loads of other nutrients, minerals, and vitamins from the assorted vegetables, which I greatly appreciate, but because of the flavor. Goodness me! Cooking chicken breast with the bone just makes it taste so much better and of course increases the nutrients. There is an old saying "the nearer the bone, the sweater the meat"; leaving the bone in adds a ton of flavor in the cooking process, a depth of flavor that you won't necessarily get from boneless chicken breast.

Place a sheet pan on a rack in the middle of the oven and preheat the oven to 425°F.

In a large bowl, stir together the maple syrup, honey, mustard, and sage. Season the chicken with a little salt and toss in the bowl to evenly coat. Carefully remove the pan from the oven. Place the chicken on the pan skin-side up and bake until the juices flow, about 20 minutes.

Meanwhile, in a large bowl, toss together the potatoes, carrots, onion, squash, Brussels sprouts, oil, ¾ teaspoon of salt, and ¾ teaspoon of pepper. When the chicken has been cooking for 20 minutes, using a pot holder, remove and carefully pour off any juices, then spread the vegetable mixture in an even layer around the chicken.

Sprinkle the chicken with ½ teaspoon of salt and ¼ teaspoon of pepper and bake until the chicken is just cooked through, 165°F on a meat thermometer, about 20 minutes more. Remove the bones from the chicken before serving and save them to make broth if you like.

NOTE: Do not serve raw honey to babies twelve months or younger, as it may cause infant botulism. Use mustard flavored with maple syrup instead.

2 tablespoons olive oil
1½ cups chopped onions
3 stalks celery, thinly sliced
2 large carrots, thinly sliced
1 pound shiitake mushrooms, sliced
8 cloves garlic, minced
2 quarts low-sodium chicken broth
2 cups cooked chickpeas, drained; if using canned, drained and rinsed
1 teaspoon grated peeled fresh ginger
4 sprigs thyme
1 small Scotch bonnet pepper or habanero (optional)
2 bay leaves
2 pounds (about 8) bone-in, skin-on chicken thighs
1½ teaspoons sea salt
½ teaspoon crushed red pepper flakes
12 ounces kale, stems removed and leaves torn

Healing Chicken Soup

This soup is highly nutritious, with plenty of immunity-enhancing ingredients, as well as collagen. But in order to get the maximum benefits, follow the recipe exactly. For instance, if you leave out the shiitake mushrooms, you won't get the same amount of vitamin B. Pasture-raised chickens contain more amino acids, including glutathione, which is so beneficial that many people take it as a supplement to reduce inflammation. The garlic is an anti-inflammatory, the veggies are rich in antioxidants, and the chickpeas have high levels of zinc. Together, the result is super tasty, super healing, and very comforting. At home we add Scotch bonnet peppers, which are similar to habaneros, to our soups for extra heat and nutrients. Give them a try if you like spicy food. You will be glad you did.

In a large Dutch oven, heat the oil over medium heat. Add the onions, celery, and carrots and cook, stirring occasionally, until the onions are translucent, about 5 minutes. Add the mushrooms and garlic and cook, stirring occasionally, for about 3 minutes more.

Add the broth, chickpeas, ginger, thyme, Scotch bonnet or habanero, if using, and bay leaves and bring to a boil over high heat. Add the chicken, salt, and red pepper flakes, reduce the heat to a simmer, and cook, covered, until the chicken is just cooked through, 165°F on a meat thermometer, about 25 minutes.

Transfer the chicken to a plate and let cool slightly. Remove the skin and bones. Discard the skin if you are using regular chicken; save the bones, or both bones and skin if using pasture-raised chicken, to make broth, if you like. Shred the meat with your hands or a fork, and place it in the pot. Add the kale, stir, and simmer, covered, until the kale is just tender, about 5 minutes. (To maintain the maximum nutrients, simmer, don't boil the kale.) Discard the thyme sprigs and bay leaves before serving.

Herb- and Parmesan-Crusted Chicken

½ cup freshly grated Parmesan cheese, preferably Parmigiano Reggiano
1 teaspoon Italian seasoning
1 teaspoon finely chopped fresh rosemary leaves
1 teaspoon finely chopped fresh thyme leaves
1 teaspoon crushed red pepper flakes
5 cloves garlic, minced
2 large boneless, skinless chicken breasts (about 1½ pounds), halved lengthwise to make 4 cutlets
1 teaspoon sea salt, or to taste
½ teaspoon freshly ground black pepper, or to taste
3 tablespoons olive oil

We don't eat a lot of dairy at home, but you can always find a block of good-quality Parmesan cheese in the refrigerator. The real Parmigiano Reggiano, a traditional hard Italian cheese, is chock-full of nutrients including calcium, magnesium, phosphorus, vitamin A, and probiotics, which are beneficial to gut health, and is naturally lactose-free. Please keep in mind it is not the same as the cheese labled "Parmesan" you find in the market in bottle shakers and bags. If you love cheese the way we do, trust me it is worth spending a little more for the real deal so you get both the amazing taste and the nutrients. A little goes a long way; my block lasts me 2 to 3 months in the refrigerator. Instead of coating my chicken breast with traditional bread coating I use my Parmigiano Reggiano. You will love this recipe and I promise you won't miss the breading. Serve with Quinoa with Cilantro and Lemon (page 242), Chickpea and Cucumber Salad (page 252), or Stir-Fried Cauliflower Rice (page 241).

In a shallow plate, stir together the cheese, Italian seasoning, rosemary, thyme, red pepper flakes, and garlic.

Season the chicken with salt and black pepper to taste, then dredge each piece in the cheese mixture, shake off any excess, and set on a large plate.

In a large skillet, heat the oil over medium-high heat. Add the chicken and cook until golden brown and just cooked through, about 3 to 4 minutes per side, flipping once.

Serve.

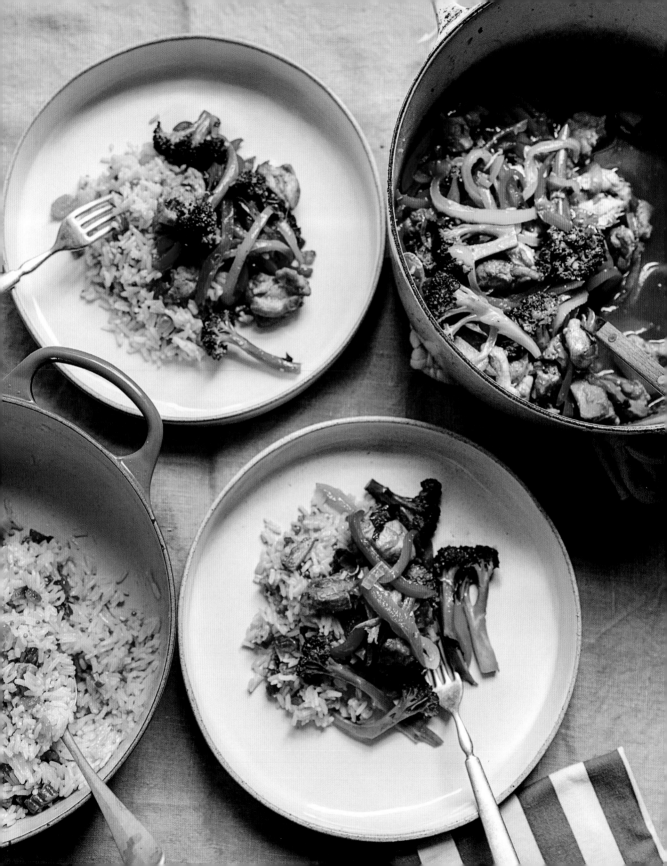

2 boneless, skinless chicken breasts, cut into 1-inch pieces
2 teaspoons curry powder
⅛ teaspoon smoked paprika
½ teaspoon sea salt
3 tablespoons olive oil, divided
1 red onion, sliced
3 cups broccoli florets
1 red bell pepper, seeded and sliced
1 yellow bell pepper, seeded and sliced
2 cloves garlic, minced
½ cup low-sodium chicken broth
2 tablespoons fresh lime juice
2 teaspoons tamari
¼ cup chopped fresh basil
2 scallions, chopped

Curried Chicken Stir-Fry

I host a lot of dinners at my home, and this fast and easy chicken stir-fry is a reliable crowd-pleaser. Depending on who is coming over, I sometimes make two batches—one with dark meat and one with white meat. (I prefer it with dark, but some of my friends only eat white chicken meat.) Curry makes everything taste and smell good, in my humble opinion, not to mention the powerful anti-inflammatory benefits it adds to food. This is a delightful dish to look at, and it tastes just as good as it looks. Serve with Quinoa with Cilantro and Lemon (page 242) or Nutty Spiced Rice (page 245).

In a large bowl, toss together the chicken, curry powder, smoked paprika, and salt.

In a large skillet, heat 1 tablespoon of the oil over medium-high heat. Add the chicken and cook, stirring occasionally, until just cooked through, about 6 minutes. Transfer the chicken to a medium bowl and set aside, reserving the skillet.

In the same skillet, heat the remaining 2 tablespoons of oil over medium-high heat. Add the onion and cook, stirring occasionally, until translucent, 4 to 5 minutes. Add the broccoli, bell peppers, and garlic and cook, stirring constantly, until the peppers are crisp-tender, about 2 minutes. Add the broth, cover, and cook until the broccoli is crisp-tender, about 4 minutes more.

Add the chicken, lime juice, and tamari and stir. Adjust the seasoning as needed. Continue cooking for about a minute more or until the chicken is heated through. Serve garnished with the basil and scallions.

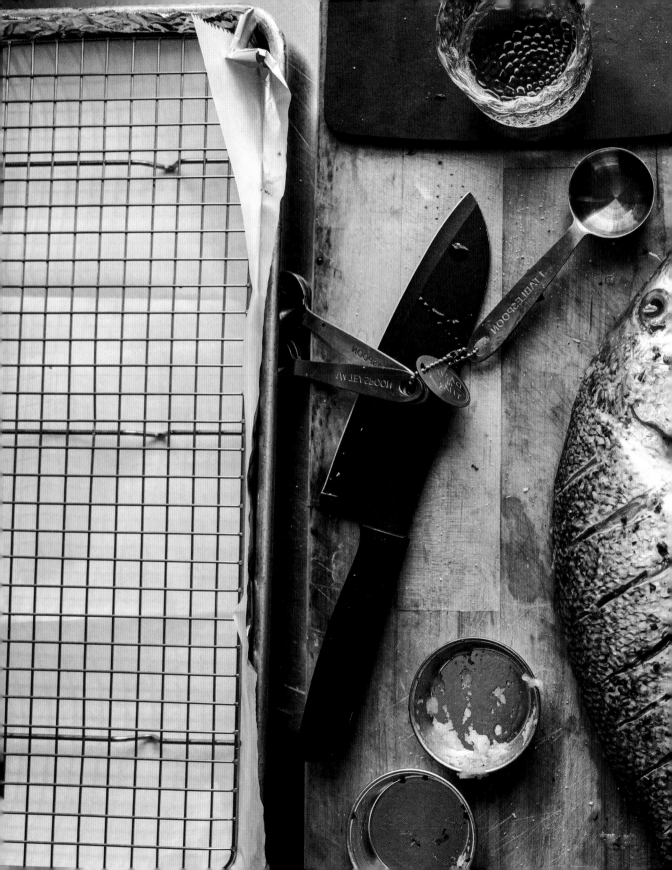

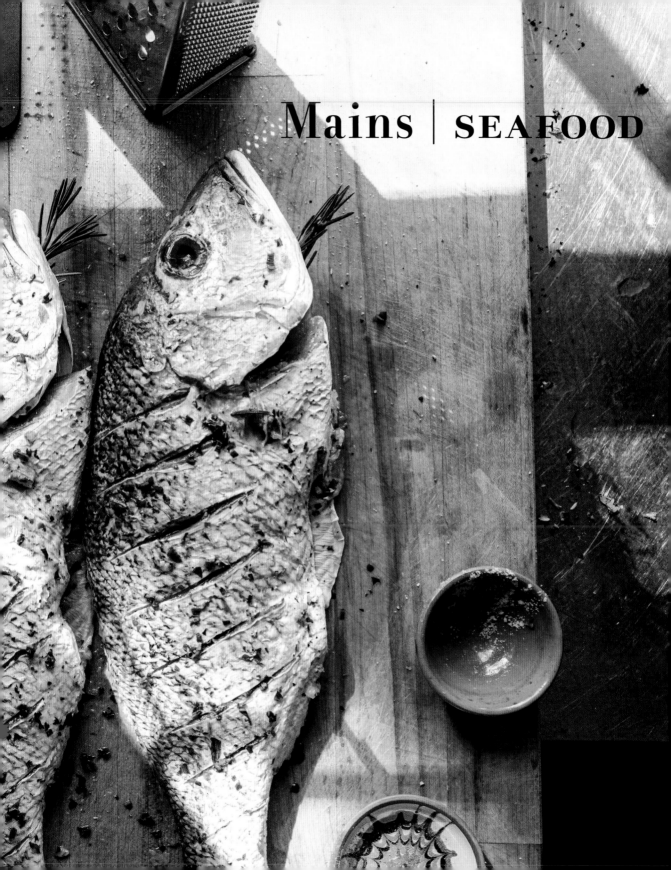

DID YOU KNOW THAT EATING seafood regularly has been shown to lower the risk of many common health problems? Fish and shellfish are the richest sources of the long-chain omega-3 fatty acids DHA and EPA, and deficiencies in those substances have been linked to cancer, depression, allergies, inflammatory diseases, cardiovascular disease, eczema, asthma, autoimmune disease, violence, dyslexia, memory problems, Alzheimer's, diabetes, and the list goes on and on. I try to eat seafood at least two times a week, and these are some of my tried-and-true recipes. But before you get cooking, it's also important to be aware of where your seafood comes from and to make informed decisions at the market.

There is a world of difference between seafood that is caught in the wild and seafood that is farm-bred or farm-raised. Farm-bred seafood have lower levels of healthy nutrients, and the hugely beneficial omega-3 fatty acids that people associate with seafood are less usable to our bodies from farm-raised specimens compared to their wild-caught counterparts. For example farm-raised fish—the most common of which are salmon, tilapia, sea bass, catfish, and cod—also have a lower protein content, and because they are confined, they tend to be fattier. I suggest that you stick to wild-caught seafood even if that means you need to limit your consumption, since it's generally pricier than farm-raised. Another consideration is being mindful of which fish are on the famed Monterey Bay Aquarium's Seafood Watch list, opting for those considered "Best Choices" (see https://www.seafoodwatch.org/).

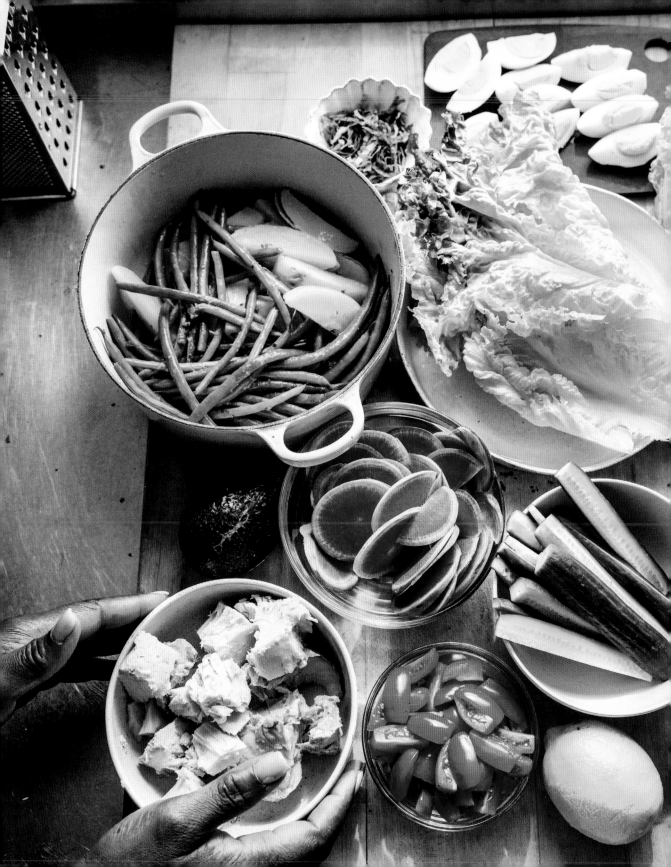

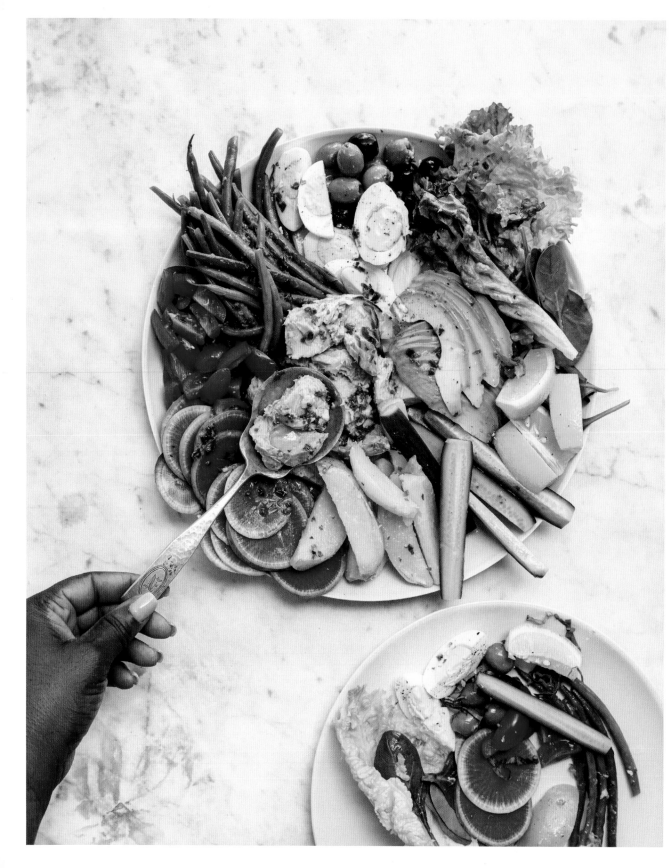

Salade Niçoise

NIÇOISE SALAD

This classic French composed salad, loaded with a variety of vegetables, is beautiful, flavorful, and very nutritious. It's also easy to prepare and great for a lazy lunch or dinner since you can make the entire thing in advance and it holds really well. Scale it up and feed a crowd—they'll be happy you did! You can use regular green beans in place of the haricots verts. Blanch them for about 3 minutes. For a vegetarian version, replace the fish with cooked chickpeas, tempeh, cauliflower "steak," or sautéed mushrooms.

For the vinaigrette, in a small bowl, whisk together all the ingredients and set aside.

For the salad, in a medium pot, combine the potatoes and enough water to cover them. Season the water with salt, bring to a boil over medium-high heat, and cook the potatoes until fork-tender, 8 to 14 minutes.

Add the haricots verts to the pot during the last 1 to 2 minutes, then drain the vegetables. When the potatoes are cool enough to handle, quarter and place them in a medium bowl with the haricots verts. Drizzle with some of the vinaigrette and toss gently.

On a large platter, arrange the fish in the center. Arrange the haricots verts, potatoes, olives, tomatoes, eggs, cucumbers, radish, leafy greens, and avocado, if using, in sections around the fish. Drizzle with the remaining vinaigrette and top with the basil. Finish with a sprinkle of salt and freshly ground black pepper, if you like, and serve.

NOTE: Do not serve raw honey to babies twelve months or younger, as it may cause infant botulism. Use maple syrup instead.

LEMON GARLIC VINAIGRETTE
⅓ cup olive oil
5 tablespoons fresh lemon juice
1 teaspoon Dijon mustard
1 clove garlic, finely minced
1 teaspoon raw honey (see Note)
½ teaspoon sea salt
2 tablespoons sliced fresh chives

SALAD
½ pound unpeeled small Yukon gold potatoes (about 4)
Sea salt
½ pound haricots verts
2 (6-ounce) cans tuna or salmon packed in olive oil, drained
1 cup mixed olives
1 cup cherry tomatoes, quartered
3 hard-boiled eggs, quartered
2 small Persian cucumbers, quartered
1 watermelon radish, thinly sliced
2 cups leafy greens (lettuce, spinach, etc.)
1 avocado, halved, peeled, pitted, and sliced (optional)
2 tablespoons roughly chopped fresh basil
Freshly ground black pepper (optional)

Cod and Vegetable Hot Pot

Hot pot has long been a favorite of mine; it is pure comfort, especially in the colder months, but do you want to know what I really love the most about this dish? Its versatility: It moves with the season and your family's preference so easily. Try switching up the vegetables with what is in season, and swap salmon for cod. The hint of smoked paprika and cumin not only adds flavor to the dish but also brings in added health benefits. Cumin is a favorite in my kitchen; it is chock-full of beneficial plant compounds, including flavonoids, and works as a wonderful digestive aid. The high level of zinc and B vitamins from the cod also leaves me feeling energized and happy. This dish is an entire meal by itself. You can, however, stretch it a little by eating it with a good piece of crusty bread.

In a medium Dutch oven, heat the oil over medium heat. Add the onion and leek and cook, stirring occasionally, until the onion is translucent, about 5 minutes. Add the garlic and cook, stirring, for about 1 minute more.

Add the tomato paste, cumin, smoked paprika, ½ teaspoon of salt, and the black pepper and stir for about 30 seconds, scraping the bottom of the pot to prevent sticking. Stir in the broth, scraping the bottom of the pot to loosen any caramelized bits, and bring to a simmer.

Add the carrots, potatoes, and Scotch bonnet pepper, if using, and simmer for 10 minutes. Add the zucchini, green beans, and ½ teaspoon of salt, stir, and cook until the vegetables are almost tender, about 10 minutes more. Gently add the fish, return the liquid to a simmer, and cook until the fish is just cooked through, 3 to 4 minutes more. Serve topped with the parsley.

---

2 tablespoons olive oil
1 onion, finely chopped
1 leek, pale green and white parts, chopped
4 cloves garlic, minced
3 tablespoons tomato paste
1½ teaspoons ground cumin
¼ teaspoon smoked paprika
1 teaspoon sea salt, divided
½ teaspoon freshly ground black pepper
4 cups low-sodium chicken broth
3 carrots, cut into 1-inch chunks
2 Yukon gold potatoes, peeled and cut into 1-inch cubes
1 small Scotch bonnet pepper or ½ teaspoon crushed red pepper flakes (optional)
2 zucchini, cut into 1-inch cubes
6 ounces green beans, halved on the bias
1½ pounds cod fillets, cut into 1½-inch chunks
¼ cup chopped fresh flat-leaf parsley

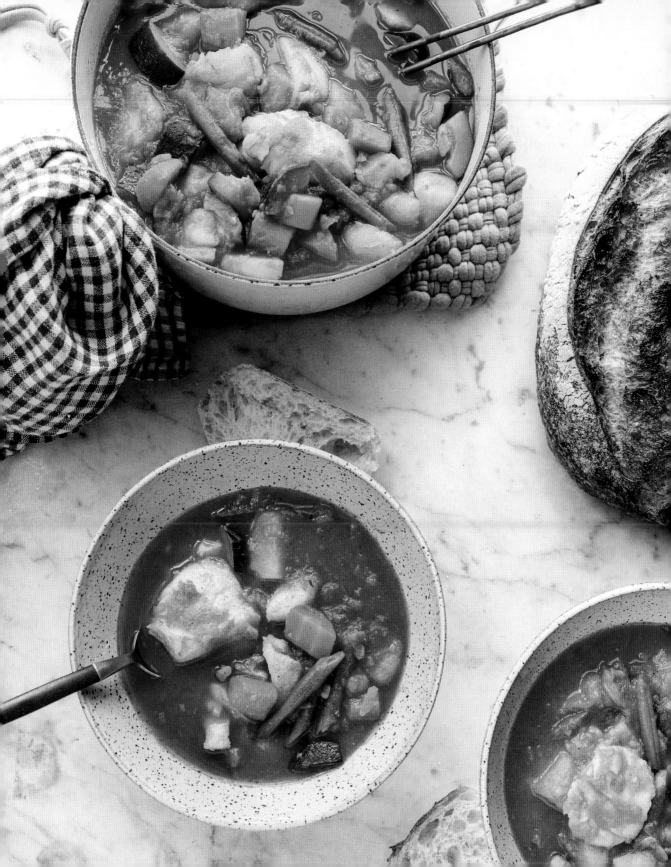

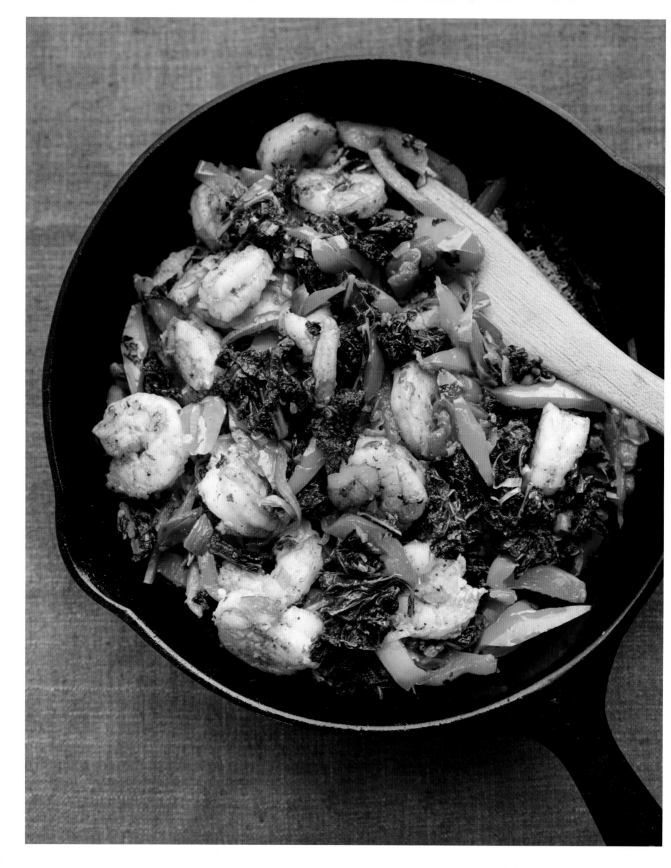

Pan-Seared Shrimp with Peppers, Tomatoes, and Kale

3 tablespoons olive oil, divided

3 cloves garlic, minced, divided

1 pound large shrimp, peeled and deveined

Sea salt

Freshly ground black pepper

1 red onion, sliced

½ leek, pale green and white parts, chopped (about ½ cup)

10 cherry tomatoes, halved

3 scallions, thinly sliced

1 yellow bell pepper, seeded and sliced

1 red bell pepper, seeded and sliced

1 teaspoon Bragg Liquid Aminos; for soy-free, use coconut aminos

2 bunches kale (about 2 pounds total), stemmed and roughly chopped

These flavors blend so beautifully, and so do the nutrients; the fat-soluble antioxidants in tomato, such as lycopene and beta-carotene, are more easily absorbed by the body when paired with olive oil. This dish also includes immunity-boosting support from the selenium and zinc that are abundant in shrimp. Not only does the dish taste good, but it is also healthy and vibrant in color. I love to blanch my kale before using it, for that extra pop of bold green. My hack with kale is to buy lots when in season, and blanch and freeze it in portion sizes for my favorite recipes—like this one. I like to serve this with Quinoa with Cilantro and Lemon (page 242).

In a medium skillet, heat 1 tablespoon of the oil over medium-high heat. Add 1 teaspoon of garlic to the skillet. Add the shrimp and salt and pepper, to taste, and cook until shrimp are pink, about 2 minutes per side, flipping once. Transfer to a plate and set aside, reserving the pan.

Add the remaining 2 tablespoons of oil to the pan and reduce the heat to medium. Add the onion and leek and cook, stirring occasionally, until the onion is translucent, about 5 minutes. Add the remaining garlic and cook, stirring, for about 1 minute more.

Add the tomatoes, scallions, and bell peppers and cook, stirring often, until the liquid is almost evaporated, about 6 minutes.

Add the aminos and kale and cook, stirring occasionally, until the kale is lightly wilted and tender, 2 to 3 minutes. Add the shrimp and any juices on the plate, stir, then season with salt and pepper as needed and serve.

Sautéed Shrimp, Vegetables, and Zucchini Noodles in a Creamy Sauce

Zoodles—spiralized zucchini noodles—are a gut-friendly, nutrient-dense, gluten-free alternative to traditional wheat pasta. No, they don't taste like pasta or have the same mouthfeel, but they are damn delicious. This dish comes together synergistically as a gut-friendly dish: every delicious bit from fiber-rich asparagus, omega-3–rich shrimp, and prebiotic-rich onions is a gift to the microbiome. It is also super creamy (despite the fact it is dairy-free), and so beautiful looking with its variety of colorful vegetables that lend texture and flavor, proving again that seriously healthy food never has to be bland or boring.

In a large skillet, heat 2 tablespoons of the oil over medium heat. Add the shrimp, add a little salt and pepper, and cook until lightly pink, about 2 minutes, turning once. Transfer to a plate, reserving the pan.

Heat the remaining 2 tablespoons of oil in the skillet. Add the onion and cook, stirring occasionally, until translucent, about 5 minutes.

Meanwhile, heat another large skillet over medium heat. Add the zucchini and ¼ teaspoon of salt and cook, covered and stirring occasionally, until crisp-tender, about 5 minutes. Drain any excess liquid from the skillet and set aside.

To the skillet with the onion, add the mushrooms, scallions, and bell peppers and cook, stirring occasionally, for about 4 minutes. Add the asparagus and cook, stirring occasionally, for about 1 minute more. Sprinkle in the flour and cook, stirring, for about 30 seconds.

Stir in the milk and garlic, followed by the peas, shrimp (along with any juice), and parsley. Cook, stirring occasionally, until the sauce thickens, about 4 minutes. (Add some broth if the sauce gets too thick.)

Remove from the heat. Add the zucchini, salt to taste, and the ½ teaspoon of pepper and toss to combine. Transfer to a serving dish and serve.

Ingredients

¼ cup olive oil, divided
1 pound large shrimp, peeled and deveined
Sea salt
½ teaspoon freshly ground black pepper, plus more to season shrimp
½ onion, thinly sliced
1½ pounds zucchini noodles (homemade or store bought; for homemade, about 4 medium zucchini)
1 cup sliced button mushrooms
4 scallions, thinly sliced
1 red bell pepper, seeded and sliced, then halved crosswise
½ pound asparagus, cut into 2-inch pieces on the bias
2 tablespoons all-purpose flour
1 cup Almond Milk (page 269) or your favorite unsweetened milk
2 large cloves garlic, finely minced
1 cup frozen peas, thawed
¼ cup minced fresh flat-leaf parsley
½ cup low-sodium chicken broth, if needed to thin the sauce

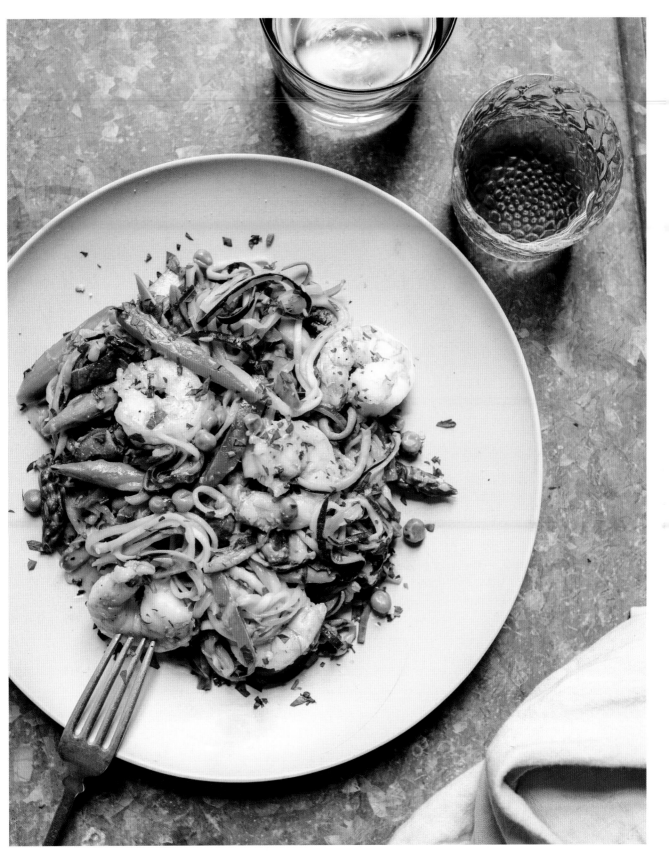

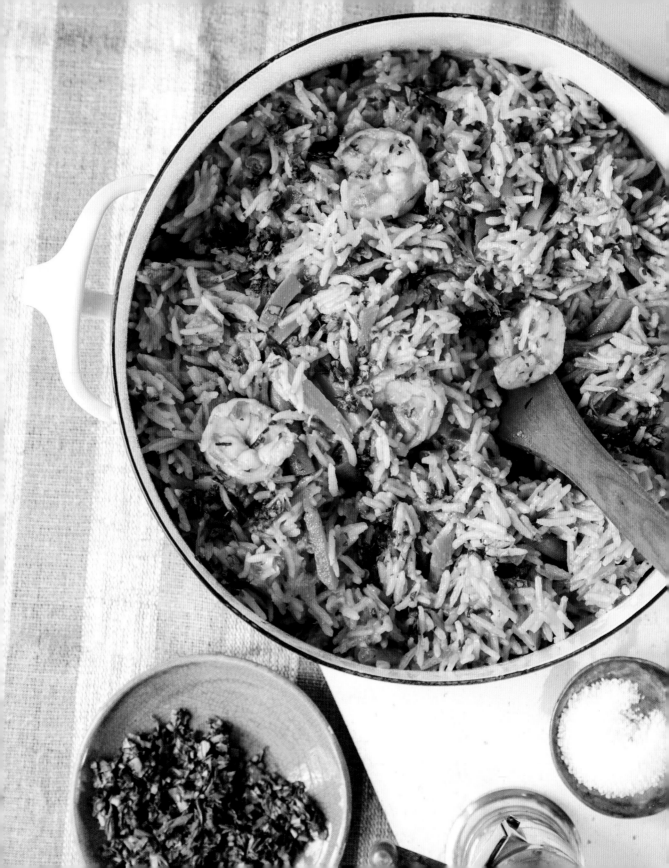

SERVES 4 TO 6

Coconut Jollof Rice

Jollof, named after the Wolof people from Senegal, is a Western/sub-Saharan African one-pot rice dish that usually contains tomatoes, seafood or meat, vegetables, and spices. You probably don't know this, but there is an active jollof "war" between Cameroonians, Nigerians, and Ghanaians, each of whom claims rights to the best-tasting version of the dish. My father is from Cameroon and my mother is from Nigeria, so I believe I have a better perspective about this than most. So, which jollof do I think is better? All of them! I suggest you start with making this Cameroonian jollof and then try the others. My guess is that you, too, will love each and every one. And here's a true story that shows how much a part of my life this dish has been: When I was growing up, there were two meals Mami would make when I wasn't feeling well, jollof and ekwang (made of freshly grated peeled cocoyam, wrapped in tiny cut cocoyam leaves, and slowly simmered in broth consisting of palm oil, smoked fish, crayfish, and traditional herbs and spices to perfection). If I turned down either she knew it was time to take me to the doctor.

In a medium pot with a tight-fitting lid, heat the coconut oil over medium-high heat. Add the onion, leeks, and bay leaf and cook, stirring occasionally, until the onion is translucent, about 5 minutes. Add the garlic and cook, stirring often, for 30 seconds more.

Add the tomato paste and tomatoes and cook, stirring occasionally, for 4 minutes. Add the coconut milk, broth, Better Than Bouillon or coconut aminos, ginger, scallions, salt, and red pepper flakes, if using, and bring to a boil. Add the rice, stir to combine, and return to a boil. Reduce the heat to medium, cover the pot, and gently simmer for 10 minutes. Add the carrots, green beans, and shrimp, mix well, re-cover the pot, and continue cooking for 5 minutes without uncovering the pot. Remove from the heat and let rest, covered, for 10 minutes. Using a fork, fluff in the basil and serve.

3 tablespoons coconut oil

1 red onion, diced

2 tablespoons thinly sliced leeks, pale green or white parts, or both

1 bay leaf

2 cloves garlic, minced

2 tablespoons tomato paste

1¼ cups chopped tomatoes

1¼ cups Coconut Milk (page 270)

1 cup low-sodium chicken broth

1 teaspoon Better Than Bouillon or coconut aminos

1 teaspoon grated peeled fresh ginger

3 scallions, thinly sliced

1 teaspoon sea salt

½ teaspoon crushed red pepper flakes or 1 small Scotch bonnet pepper (optional)

1½ cups basmati rice, rinsed until the water runs clear

2 small carrots, cut into ½-inch dice (1 cup)

8 ounces green beans, cut into 1-inch pieces

1 pound large shrimp, peeled, deveined, and rinsed

¼ cup finely chopped fresh basil

Shrimp and Tomato Stew with Scallions

¼ cup olive oil
1 onion, chopped
2 cloves garlic, minced
3 cups (4 medium) tomatoes, diced
¾ cup dry white wine
1 teaspoon dried oregano
1½ teaspoons sea salt
1 small Scotch bonnet pepper, or ½ teaspoon crushed red pepper flakes (optional)
1¾ pounds large shrimp, shelled and deveined
4 scallions, thinly sliced
¼ teaspoon freshly ground black pepper
¼ cup chopped fresh flat-leaf parsley, divided

I love just about any kind of seafood, especially shrimp. With a little inspiration from my Cameroonian roots I pulled together this little number. There is something about shrimp in stewed tomato that makes the flavors blend so well. Add scallion and oregano to the mix, and they take it to another level. All I can say is this dish just wins in taste and nutrients. All the many nutrients include protein (shrimp), and antioxidants and phytonutrients (dried oregano). Seriously, you can serve this with just about everything, including my Quinoa with Cilantro and Lemon (page 242), Stir-Fried Cauliflower Rice (page 241), or the Nutty Spiced Rice (page 245).

In a medium pot, heat the oil over medium-low heat. Add the onion and cook, stirring occasionally, until translucent, about 5 minutes. Add the garlic and cook, stirring, for about 30 seconds more.

Raise the heat to medium, add the tomatoes with their juices, and cook, stirring occasionally, for about 5 minutes. Add the wine, oregano, salt, and Scotch bonnet pepper, if using. Bring to a boil over high heat, then reduce the heat and simmer, partially covered and stirring occasionally, until thickened, about 20 minutes.

Stir in the shrimp, scallions, and pepper and simmer, covered, until the shrimp are just done, about 2 minutes. Stir in 3 tablespoons of the parsley. Serve topped with the remaining 1 tablespoon of parsley.

Creamy Salmon with Kale and Tomatoes

4 (6-ounce) salmon steaks
Sea salt
Freshly ground black pepper
3 tablespoons olive oil, divided
1 small onion, diced
4 cloves garlic, minced
⅓ cup low-sodium chicken or vegetable broth
½ cup diced tomatoes
1¾ cups Cashew Milk (see page 272)
3 packed cups stemmed and roughly chopped kale
⅓ cup freshly grated Parmesan cheese, preferably Parmigiano Reggiano
1 tablespoon chopped fresh flat-leaf parsley

This recipe shows off the incredible flavor of bone-in fish, not to mention the nutrients it lends to the dish. The creaminess of this sauce is proof you can incorporate nut milk into your meals and get the same creaminess you would with heavy cream. I love the abundance of nutrients in this dish from the omega-3 fatty acids and a host of other vitamins and minerals. The Parmigiano Reggiano takes flavor a notch higher while adding beneficial probiotics. This dish is not only delicious but it is also as healthy as they come. This dish pairs well with Stir-Fried Cauliflower Rice (page 241), Nutty Spiced Rice (page 245), a good piece of crusty bread, or whatever you like.

Season the salmon with salt and pepper. In a large skillet, heat 2 tablespoons of the oil over medium-high heat. Add the salmon and cook until almost cooked through, about 5 minutes per side, flipping once. (You can cook the fish less or more, depending on your preference and the thickness of your steak.) Transfer the fish to a plate, reserving the skillet.

Add the remaining tablespoon of oil to the fat in the skillet. Add the onion and cook, stirring occasionally, for about 2 minutes. Add the garlic and cook, stirring, for about 1 minute more. Add the broth and deglaze the skillet, scraping the bottom of the pan with a spoon to remove any caramelized bits, until the liquid is reduced slightly.

Stir in the tomatoes and cook until they break down and release their juices, about 3 minutes. Add the cashew milk, then reduce the heat so the mixture gently simmers. Add the kale, stir, and cook just until wilted, about 1 minute.

Add the cheese and stir. Taste and adjust the seasoning with salt and pepper, if necessary. Gently add the fish and any juice on the plate and let simmer for 1 minute or until heated through. Sprinkle with the parsley and serve.

2 tablespoons low-sodium chicken broth
1 tablespoon plus 1½ teaspoons fresh lemon juice, plus more for serving
1 tablespoon olive oil
1 tablespoon sriracha
2 (4-ounce) salmon fillets
Sea salt
Freshly ground black pepper
1 pound medium-thick asparagus
4 cloves garlic, minced
4 scallions, thinly sliced on the bias
2 tablespoons chopped fresh flat-leaf parsley

Salmon and Asparagus en Papillote

I grew up eating mpuh fish, a traditional fish dish steamed in plantain leaves. I thought the plantain leaf was the secret sauce because the mpuh fish tasted so good; little did I know it was because of the cooking process, not the leaves. Cooking en papillote is a method that involves sealing food in a packet (papillote) made of a leaf, parchment paper, or aluminum foil. The fish, along with your herbs and vegetables, are sealed in the papillote and then baked or steamed, as we do in Cameroon. This dish checks all of my top three Bs: presentation benefit, health benefit, and taste benefit. Listen, this is such a game-changing way to cook fast, healthy meals with no pots and pans to clean, and an easy way to make an impressive dish. Just place your ingredients in parchment paper, seal, pop in the oven, and let the steam in the papillote do its thing. I love this dish for many obvious reasons and hope you do, too. Don't stop with this dish though; explore more ways to cook en papillote. Try shrimp, potatoes, and more.

Preheat the oven to 425°F. Cut two 14 × 12–inch pieces of parchment paper into large heart shapes, then fold in half from side to side to make a crease, open the hearts, and set aside.

In a small bowl, combine the broth, lemon juice, olive oil, and sriracha and set aside.

Season the salmon with salt and pepper and set each piece lengthwise on one half of each parchment heart. Lay half of the asparagus lengthwise next to each piece of salmon and sprinkle with a little salt. (Do not oversalt.) Scatter the garlic and scallions on top, then drizzle with the broth mixture.

Close the hearts by folding the empty half of each heart over the ingredients and crimping the edges of the two halves together in small overlapping folds until completely sealed. Do not wrap too tightly, though; you need a little space inside for the heat to circulate. Twist the end of each packet so no juice or steam runs out during baking.

(Continued)

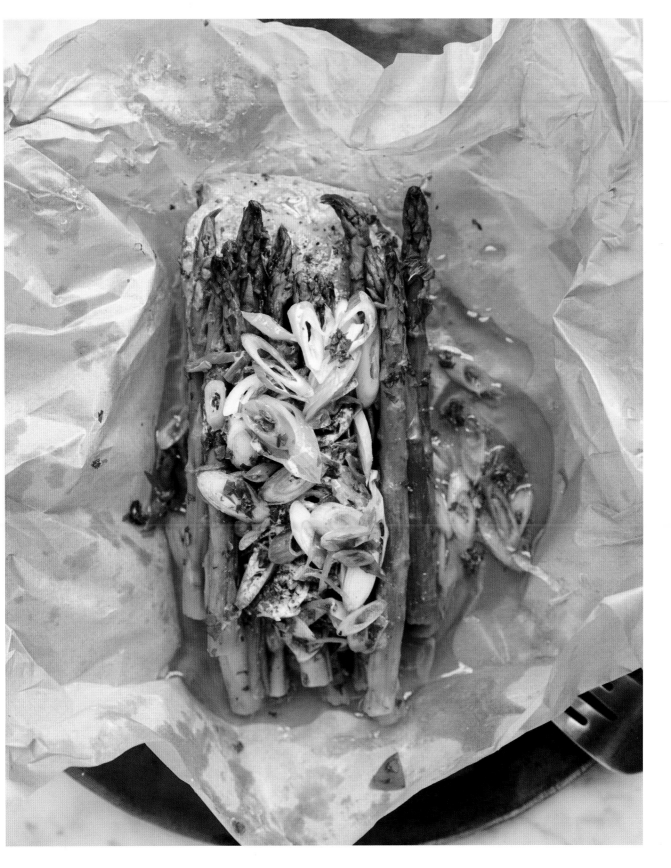

Transfer the packets to a sheet pan and bake until the salmon has just cooked through, 9 to 12 minutes. (Test one packet; if the salmon isn't done, reseal as best you can and continue baking a little longer.) Let rest for about 2 minutes.

Transfer the packets to two plates, cut or tear open the center of each, and garnish with the parsley and more lemon juice, if you like. Serve.

Who knew boosting your immunity could be as simple as eating more garlic? According to the Iowa Women's Health Study involving 41,000 women between the ages of 55 and 69, those who routinely ate garlic (and fruits and vegetables) had a 35 percent lower risk for colon cancer than those who did not. Garlic is chock-full of healing compounds, including allium and quercetin, which have antiviral and antibiotic properties. Food truly can be medicine when consumed properly.

2 tablespoons olive
  oil, plus more for
  greasing the broiler
  rack
1 teaspoon fresh
  thyme leaves
Juice of ½ lemon
4 (6- to 8-ounce) tuna
  steaks
Sea salt
Freshly ground black
  pepper
4 tomatoes, seeded
  and diced
Kernels from 2 ears of
  cooked corn on the
  cob
1 onion, finely chopped
1 red bell pepper,
  seeded and diced
1 cup chopped fresh
  cilantro
2 limes

Tuna Steaks
with Tomato and Corn Salsa

Where I grew up, on the coastline of the Atlantic Ocean in Cameroon, West Africa, seafood was and still is a predominate dish. To this day you can go to the beachside in Limbe (formerly Victoria) and eat some of the tastiest and freshest roasted seafood ever. Fast-forward to a working trip to Puerto Rico, I tried ceviche for the very first time. Oh my word, the explosion of flavors in my mouth! That might have been my very first time eating raw fish. The African in me was surprised I enjoyed it so much.

This recipe is my way to enjoy cooked tuna but with an explosion of flavors so all my non-raw-fish-eating family members can enjoy it, too. I love the jazzy flavors of the tomato and corn salsa. Don't be tempted to make it with frozen corn. It's worth waiting until fresh corn is in season. For a smoky twist, roast the corn instead of boiling it. And if you want to take this a notch higher, add some Scotch bonnet pepper (or habanero), as we do in my kitchen, or take baby steps by adding seeded, diced jalapeño pepper to the delicious salsa. This dish is both flavorful and nutritious.

In a shallow dish large enough to hold the tuna steaks, stir together the oil, thyme, and lemon juice. Season the tuna with salt and pepper, then place it in the dish and turn until thoroughly coated with the marinade. Cover and refrigerate for 1 to 2 hours, turning occasionally.

Meanwhile, make the salsa. In a medium bowl, combine the tomatoes, corn, onion, bell pepper, cilantro, juice of 1 lime, ¾ teaspoon of salt, and ¼ teaspoon of pepper. Stir, then let stand for about 1 hour at room temperature, so the flavors can blend.

Preheat the broiler, with a rack about 3 inches from the heat. Brush a broiler rack set in a broiler pan with oil. Place the tuna steaks on the rack and brush with the marinade in the dish. Broil the steaks until medium-rare, 3 to 4 minutes, turning once. (Cook them less or more, if you prefer.) Slice the second lime and serve along with the salsa.

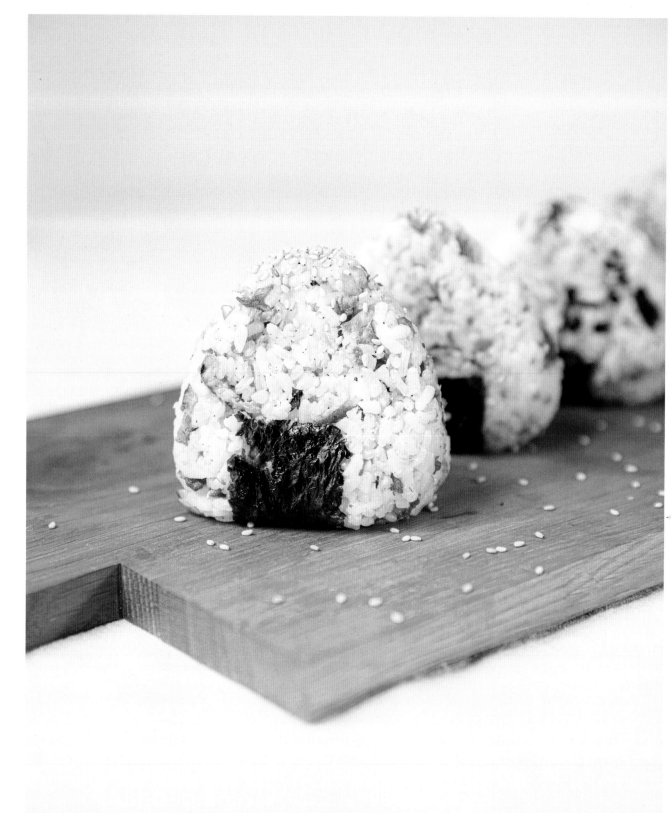

1 teaspoon olive oil
1 (8-ounce) boneless, skinless salmon fillet
1 tablespoon soy sauce
2 cups Japanese short-grain rice, cooked according to the package instructions
1½ teaspoons toasted sesame seeds, plus more for garnish
2 scallions, finely chopped
Sea salt
Two 7½ × 8–inch sheets nori, each cut lengthwise into 6 strips, then each strip folded lengthwise and cut in half

Sake Onigiri

SALMON JAPANESE RICE BALLS

The simplicity of these dried-seaweed-covered rice balls compared to the explosion of flavor they provide is mind blowing. And I especially love that they are bursting with nutrients. Did you know that nori (dried seaweed) offers one of the broadest range of nutrients of any food? Those nutrients include calcium, copper, iron, magnesium, manganese, phosphorus, potassium, selenium, zinc, and more. Nori can actually contain up to ten times more calcium than milk, and is packed full of vitamins! After you cook the rice, the onigiri take only a few minutes to prepare. They make a great snack or portable lunch, too. Dip them into soy sauce, if you like.

Heat a small skillet with the oil over medium-high heat. Add the salmon and cook, flipping once about halfway through, until cooked through 6 to 8 minutes. Using a spatula, break up the salmon into flakes in the skillet with the heat still on. Add the soy sauce, mix with the salmon flakes, and cook until the liquid is gone, 1 to 2 minutes. Transfer the salmon to a large bowl.

Fluff the cooked rice and add it to the bowl along with the sesame seeds and scallions. Mix until the salmon, sesame seeds, and scallions are evenly distributed throughout the rice.

Wet your hands with water so that the rice won't stick, then place a little salt on them and rub it all over your wet palms.

Scoop about ½ cup of the warm rice mixture into one palm and, using both hands, quickly roll it into a ball, then gently shape it into a triangle (don't squeeze it too hard) to form an onigiri. Wrap the onigiri with a piece of nori and set it on a large plate. Repeat with the remaining rice mixture and nori. Sprinkle some more sesame seeds on the finished onigiri and serve warm, at room temperature, or cold.

NOTES: For your little ones, make smaller balls. If you are not eating them immediately, it's okay to make onigiri and then add the nori just before serving so it doesn't get soggy.

Lemony Salmon Kebabs

Sometimes I just get a yearning for salmon that is really tasty but light and refreshing. If you can use wild-caught salmon here, you will be amazed at the taste. Lemon is one of my all-time favorite ingredients; it helps give these kebabs a light, smoky, citrusy finish. This is one recipe that I make year-round, either out on the grill or indoors using my grill pan. Make these for lunch or dinner—whenever you do, you'll be amazed that something that melts in your mouth is made with such ease. I like to pair the kebabs with my Nutty Spiced Rice (page 245) or Kale Salad (page 249) to make it a complete meal. Get ready because these kebabs are about to become your new favorite thing.

2 tablespoons olive oil, plus more for greasing the skillet or grill pan, if using
1 tablespoon fresh lemon juice
¼ cup finely chopped fresh flat-leaf parsley
3 cloves garlic
½ teaspoon sea salt
¼ teaspoon freshly ground black pepper
1 (1½-pound) skinless salmon fillet, cut into 1½-inch cubes

In a large bowl, stir together the oil, lemon juice, parsley, garlic, salt, and pepper. Add the salmon and gently toss until completely coated with the marinade, then thread the cubes onto the skewers.

Preheat a grill to medium. You'll need 4 long or 8 short skewers, soaked in water for at least 30 minutes if using bamboo or wood. You can also cook the kebabs in a skillet or grill pan on the stovetop with a little olive oil over medium heat, or broil them.

Grill the kebabs until just cooked through, about 8 minutes, flipping once halfway through. Serve.

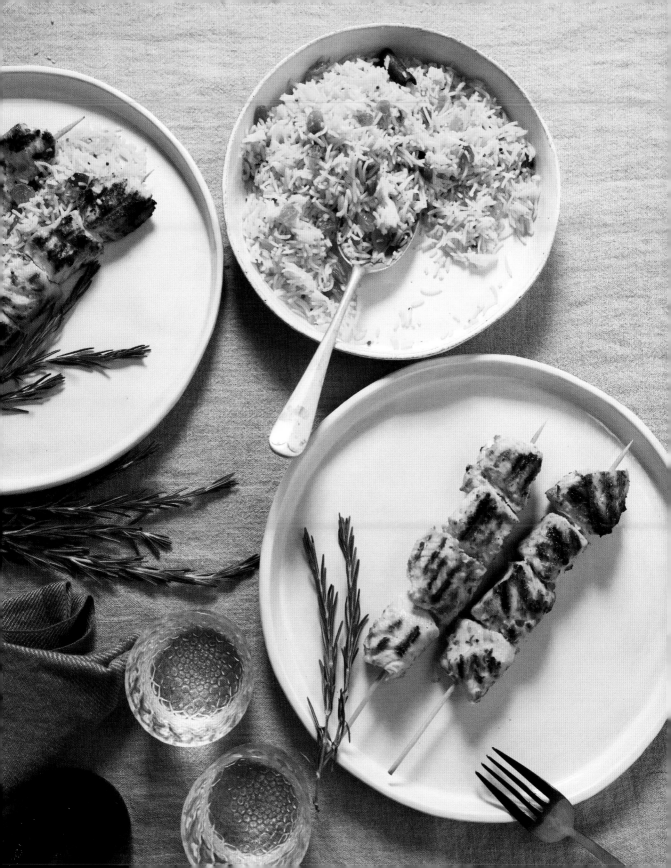

Red Snapper with Lemony Tomato Vinaigrette

This dish never fails to impress: The plated fish looks like you spent all day in the kitchen, though it is ready in a fairly short amount of time (especially if the kiddos are old enough to add their extra hands). Red snapper is especially high in potassium and rich in vitamin B$_{12}$; while nutrients are important, taste is paramount and this baby is so moist and tasty, especially if you are lucky enough to get a really fresh snapper. If you have never tasted a piece of fish from a whole roasted snapper, you are in for a pleasant surprise. When we are done eating, I throw all the bones in a pot with some water and any leftover vegetable scraps (I keep a continuous stash in my freezer) and make fish broth. Enjoy with Plantain Tapé (page 255) or Kale Salad (page 249). I grew up eating fish grilled over charcoal, and there is nothing better. If you have a charcoal grill, try cooking the snapper on it. Be sure to get the coals nice and hot and oil the grates. It should take about 7 minutes per side. Do not attempt to turn the fish until the skin has browned and crisped or it will stick.

For the fish, place the snapper on a parchment-lined sheet pan or a wire-rack on a sheet pan and make three or four shallow diagonal cuts on each side (do not cut all the way through to the bone), season with the salt and pepper, and make sure they get inside the slits. Set aside.

In a small bowl, stir together the remaining fish ingredients, except the rosemary sprigs and lemon slices, to make the marinade. Adjust the taste as needed. Rub half of the marinade all over the fish, including the cavity and slits. Cover with plastic wrap and set aside for no longer than 30 minutes while you heat the oven and make the vinaigrette. (Of course, if you need more time, be sure to refrigerate the fish.)

Preheat the oven to 450°F, with a rack in the highest position.

For the vinaigrette, in a small bowl, combine all the ingredients and gently mix together. Adjust the taste as needed, then set aside.

FISH

- 1 whole red snapper (about 2 pounds), scaled and gutted
- 1 teaspoon sea salt
- ½ teaspoon freshly ground black pepper
- ¼ cup olive oil, plus more if needed
- 2 cloves garlic, finely minced
- 2 scallions, thinly sliced
- 2 teaspoons finely chopped fresh thyme leaves
- 1 teaspoon Better Than Bouillon or coconut aminos (optional)
- ½ teaspoon ground white pepper
- 2 large sprigs rosemary
- ½ lemon, sliced

LEMONY TOMATO VINAIGRETTE

- 1 small red onion, finely diced
- 3 tablespoons white wine vinegar
- 1 tablespoon plus 2 teaspoons fresh lemon juice
- ½ teaspoon sea salt
- 3 or 4 tomatoes, diced (about 2 cups)
- ⅓ cup chopped fresh flat-leaf parsley
- ½ teaspoon grated peeled fresh ginger (optional)
- ¼ teaspoon freshly ground black pepper
- 1 small Scotch bonnet pepper (optional)

Place the rosemary sprigs and lemon slices inside the fish and roast on the top shelf until the flesh is firm when prodded with a finger, 20 to 25 minutes. Turn on the broiler, baste the fish with the remaining marinade and a little more oil if needed, and broil until lightly browned on top, 3 to 5 minutes. Let rest for about 5 minutes, then transfer to a platter. Serve with the vinaigrette.

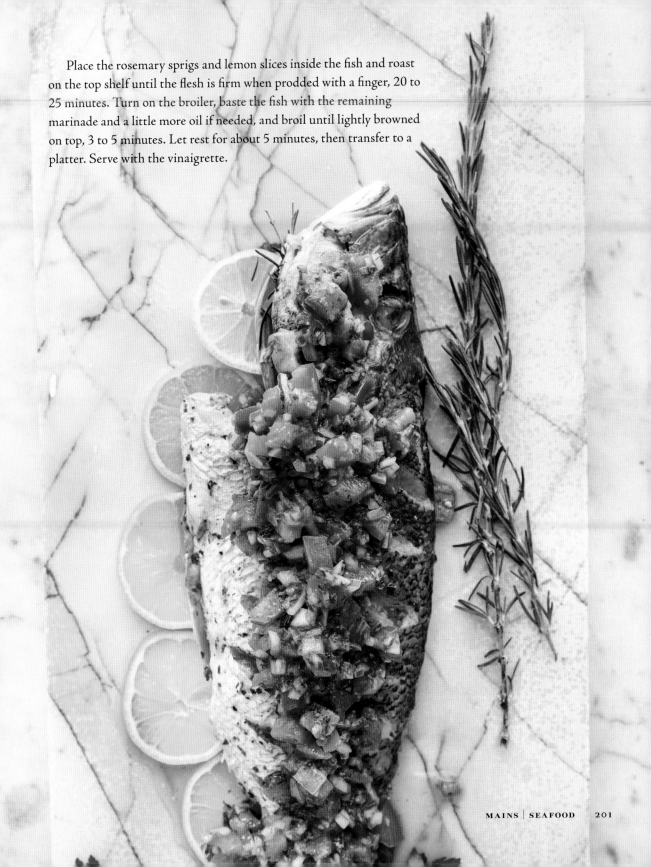

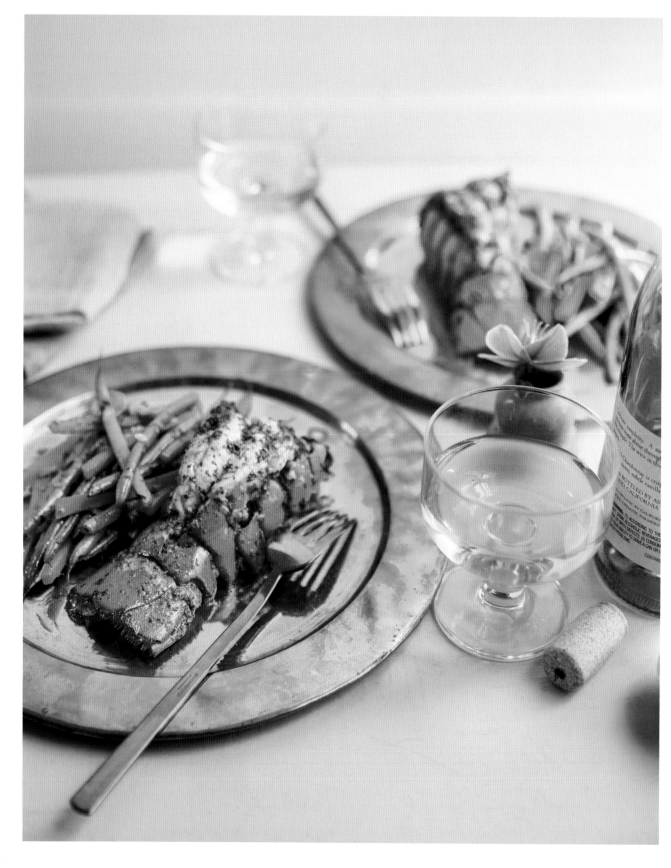

Broiled Lobster
with Fragrant Herbs

GF

SERVES 4

4 unshelled (10- to 12-ounce) lobster tails, thawed, if frozen, and rinsed
4 tablespoons (½ stick) salted butter, melted
3 cloves garlic, finely minced
2 tablespoons finely chopped fresh flat-leaf parsley
1 tablespoon finely chopped fresh thyme leaves
½ teaspoon finely chopped fresh rosemary leaves
2 teaspoons fresh lemon juice
¼ teaspoon smoked paprika
¼ teaspoon cayenne pepper (optional)
½ teaspoon sea salt
¼ teaspoon freshly ground black pepper

A few years ago, a friend wanted to re-create one of her husband's favorite experiences for their anniversary dinner but it was too expensive. She just didn't have the budget to indulge at a restaurant, let alone afford a lobster dish there. We were able to recreate her hubby's special dish for their anniversary dinner at home. This recipe is for all of us, my friend Lilly, you, and me. We can have a lavish, scrumptious restaurant-style feast for our special moment at home. And while it seems like a luxury, did you know that lobster is actually a little more nutritious than shrimp? It has more omega-3, a little more protein, and less cholesterol. If you can figure how to quickly butterfly your lobster tail this dish is a breeze to make. Thyme and rosemary not only add flavor, but they also boost the nutritional profile of the dish, and the subtle hit of smoked paprika adds a beautiful flavor and color to the lobster. Serve with Sautéed Green Beans and Carrots (page 253) and Plantain Tapé (page 255), if you like.

Preheat the broiler, with a rack 4 to 6 inches from the heat.

Butterfly the lobster shells using good kitchen scissors: Cut down the center of the top of the shell lengthwise, starting from the head end and continuing down until you reach the tail, but without cutting the tail meat. Use your thumbs to pull open the top of the shell, then gently scoop the lobster meat upward, disconnecting it from the bottom of the shell except for at the tail end. Slightly push together the empty shell underneath the meat so that the meat rests on top of the shell. Place the tails on a sheet pan.

In a small bowl, whisk together the melted butter, garlic, herbs, lemon juice, smoked paprika, cayenne, if using, salt, and black pepper. Brush the mixture on the lobster meat, then broil until the meat is just cooked through, opaque and lightly browned, about 1 minute per ounce. (For example, a 12-ounce lobster tail should take about 12 minutes.)

Serve and enjoy.

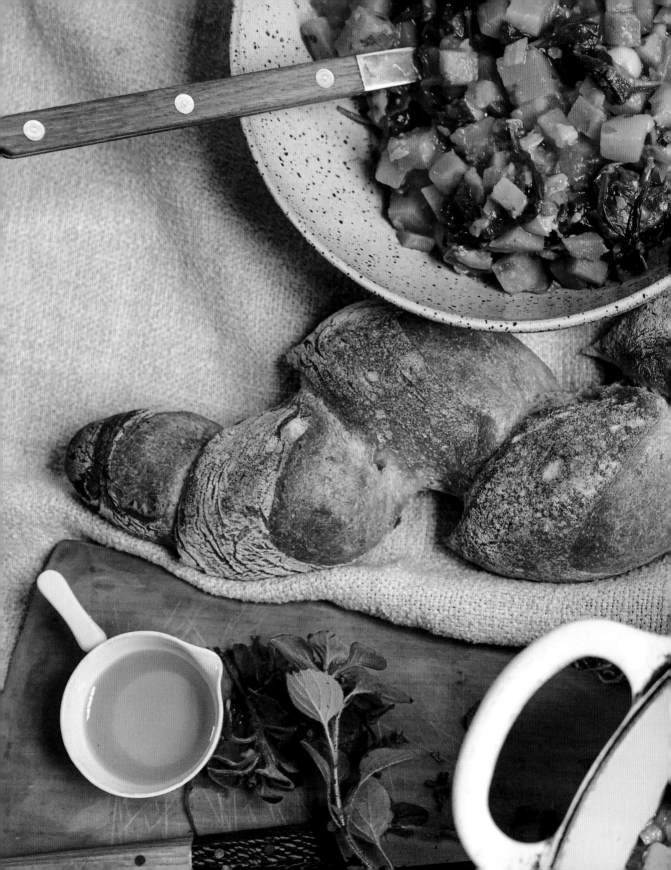

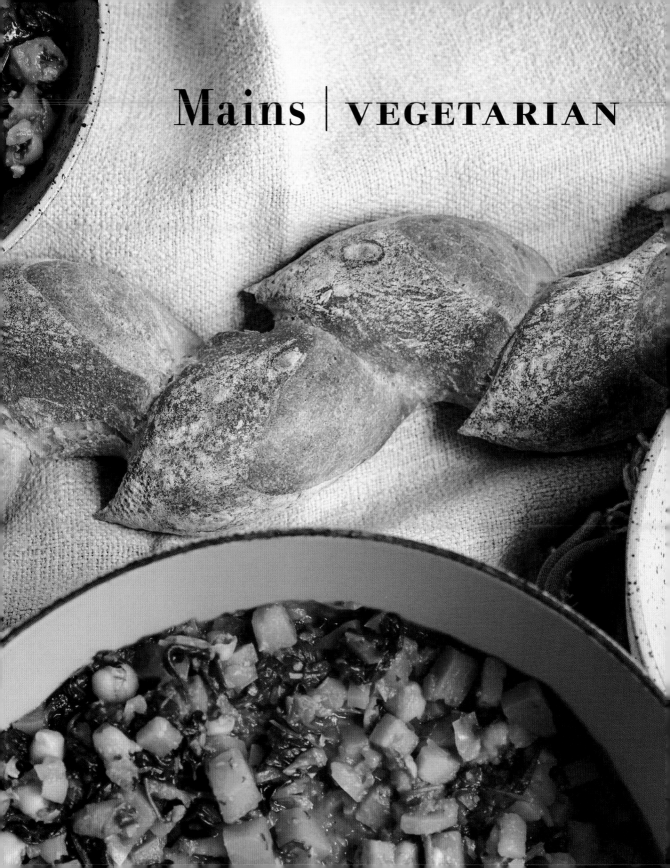

Mains | VEGETARIAN

WE ARE ALL BIOLOGICALLY different and, therefore, react differently to foods because of how our digestive and immune systems work. That said, we can all benefit from adding more plants to our diets. A diet rich in vegetables and fruits can lower blood pressure, reduce the risk of heart disease and stroke, prevent some types of cancer, lower risk of eye and digestive problems, and have a positive effect on blood sugar, which can help keep our appetite in check. Eating nonstarchy vegetables, such as leafy greens, and fruits may even promote weight loss due to their low glycemic loads.

At least nine different families of vegetables and fruits exist, each with potentially hundreds of different plant compounds that are beneficial to health. I always suggest eating a variety of types and colors of produce in order to ensure your body gets a greater diversity of beneficial plant chemicals. But that also makes it easier to create interesting, visually appealing meals. I hope this section helps you eat more life-healing plants. Every time someone tells me they hate vegetables because they taste like "dirt" a part of me wants to reach out and give them a hug because I, too, have tasted vegetables that tasted just like that. But that is not how vegetables should taste at all! Take it from someone who eats vegetables just because. At a time in my life when I eat food simply for taste and nothing else, plants are my favorite foods because of their delicious taste and vibrant colors. If you are already a vegetable fan, these recipes will make a wonderful addition to your rotation; if you, like many others, have had bad experiences with vegetables, here is another opportunity to give them another try. Black Bean Burgers (page 210) will make you a fan of plant-forward meals immediately, and the Soy-Marinated Tofu Kebabs with Pineapple and Vegetables (page 209) tastes just as good as it looks. And if you have never had beans and fresh corn stewed in a tomato base, you are in for a special treat with the Black Bean and Corn Stew (page 222). Eat for the taste, and let the abundance of nutrients be an added bonus!

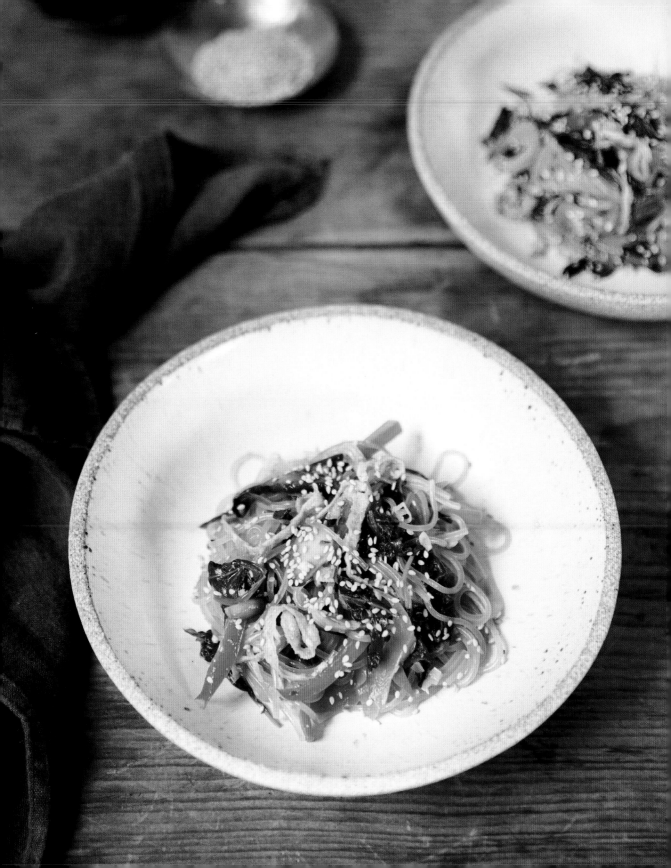

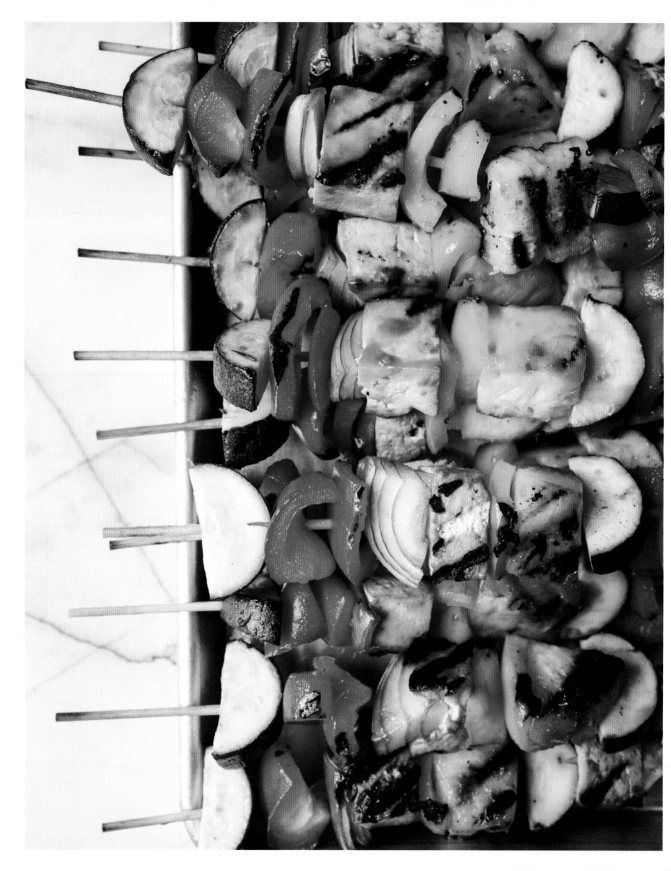

Soy-Marinated Tofu Kebabs with Pineapple and Vegetables

GF, DF

SERVES 4 TO 6

½ cup tamari
½ cup freshly squeezed orange juice
2 tablespoons maple syrup
1 teaspoon onion powder
2 cloves garlic, minced
1 teaspoon arrowroot powder
1 (14-ounce) package extra-firm tofu, drained, pressed (see sidebar, page 86), and cut into 1-inch cubes
1 red onion, quartered vertically, then halved horizontally
1 red bell pepper, seeded and cut into 1¼-inch dice
1 yellow bell pepper, seeded and cut into 1¼-inch dice
1 small zucchini, halved lengthwise and cut into 1¼-inch slices
½ pineapple, the flesh cut into 1-inch cubes
1 tablespoon olive oil
½ teaspoon salt
¼ teaspoon freshly ground black pepper

If you are on the fence about tofu, this is a wonderful "starter" recipe. These kebabs are packed with juicy sweetness and vitamin C. You can assemble these ahead of time and keep them in the fridge, covered, until you're ready to cook them. Look for sprouted organic tofu that is made from sprouted soybeans; the sprouting process makes it more digestible while improving its nutrients. Serve with Nutty Spiced Rice (page 245) or Quinoa with Cilantro and Lemon (page 242), if you like.

In a small saucepan, bring the tamari, orange juice, maple syrup, onion powder, and garlic to a boil over high heat, then reduce the heat and simmer the marinade for 1 minute.

Meanwhile, in a small bowl, mix together the arrowroot powder with 1 teaspoon water until smooth. Whisk the mixture into the marinade and cook until it thickens, about 1 minute more. Remove from the heat, cover, and let cool for about 5 minutes.

In a medium high-sided dish, combine the tofu and ⅓ to ½ cup of the marinade, then gently turn the tofu to coat all sides. Refrigerate, covered, for at least 1 hour or up to 4 hours. Reserve the remaining marinade.

Preheat a grill over medium heat. You'll need 6 long skewers, soaked in water for at least 30 minutes if using bamboo or wood.

In a large bowl, toss together the onion, peppers, zucchini, pineapple, oil, salt, and pepper. Remove the tofu from the marinade and stir that marinade into the reserved marinade in the saucepan.

Assemble the skewers in the following order: a piece of zucchini, red pepper, onion, tofu, yellow pepper, pineapple. Repeat one or two more times. Brush with a little of the marinade and grill, turning occasionally, until the tofu is slightly charred and vegetables are crisp-tender, about 8 minutes. (Brush with a little more marinade while cooking, as you like. You can also cook the kebabs a little longer if you prefer more tender vegetables.) Serve.

Black Bean Burgers

3 cups cooked black beans, drained and patted dry; if using canned, drained, rinsed, and patted dry
Extra-virgin olive oil
1 cup finely chopped onions
½ cup finely diced button mushrooms
3 cloves garlic, minced
¾ cup finely chopped red bell peppers
½ cup fresh or frozen corn; if frozen, thawed and drained
2 large eggs
½ cup bread crumbs or oat flour
2 tablespoons ketchup
1 tablespoon Worcestershire sauce
1½ teaspoons ground cumin
1 teaspoon chili powder
¼ teaspoon smoked paprika
Pinch sea salt
Freshly ground black pepper

If you're looking for an alternative to commercial high-protein, plant-based burgers, which often include ingredients you can't pronounce, try this recipe. There's nothing artificial about it, and there are no additives or fillers. And I can't even begin to explain the explosion of flavors you get with each bite. These burgers—made with black beans, bell peppers, corn, bread crumbs, and spices—are in heavy rotation in our home for both their incredible taste and their nutrients. Black beans are loaded with fiber, potassium, folate, and protein. We eat a lot of beans in our home; they are so much cheaper than chicken, beef, or fish, which are the first things I cut off my grocery list when I have a cash crunch. Looking for a meal that can fill you and your family up at an affordable price? Look no further than this wallet-friendly dish. Serve these burgers on buns with the toppings of your choice and a side of Herbed Parmesan French Fries (page 258).

Preheat the oven to 325°F. Line a baking sheet with parchment paper.

Spread the beans evenly onto the prepared sheet pan and bake until slightly dried out, about 15 minutes.

Meanwhile, in a large skillet, heat 1 tablespoon of oil over medium heat. Add the onions and cook, stirring occasionally, until translucent, about 5 minutes. Add the mushrooms and garlic and cook, stirring, for 1 minute more. Add the bell peppers and corn and cook, stirring occasionally, until tender, about 5 minutes more, then set aside.

In a large bowl, whisk the eggs, then stir in the bread crumbs, ketchup, Worcestershire sauce, cumin, chili powder, smoked paprika, salt, pepper, and the sautéed vegetables. Add the beans and mash lightly with a fork (do not overmash). Form into 8 large patties, using about ½ cup of the mixture for each or smaller for the kiddos.

In the same skillet, heat 1 tablespoon of oil over medium heat. Carefully add the patties and cook until browned and heated through, about 10 minutes, flipping once halfway through. Serve.

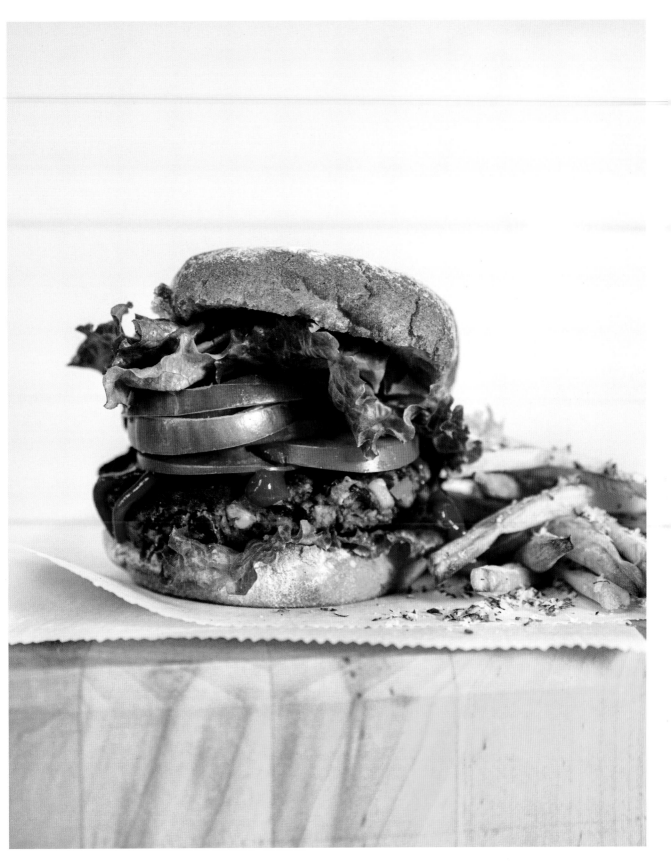

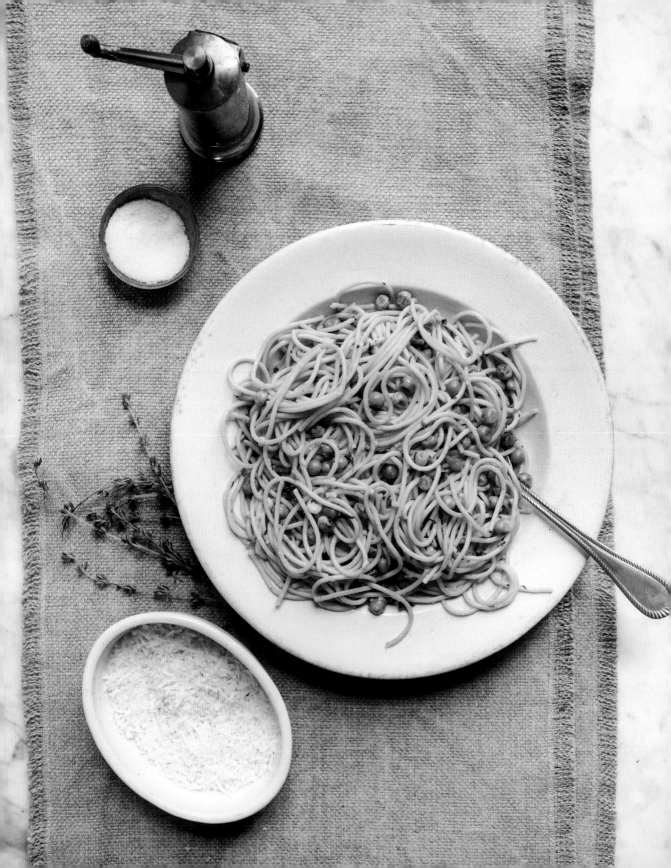

1 pound chickpea linguine
3 tablespoons olive oil, divided
4 cloves garlic, thinly sliced
1 teaspoon chopped fresh thyme leaves
Zest of 1 lemon
⅓ cup fresh lemon juice
1½ cups frozen peas, thawed
2 scallions, thinly sliced
1 teaspoon sea salt
⅛ teaspoon freshly ground black pepper
⅓ cup freshly grated Parmesan cheese, preferably Parmigiano Reggiano (optional)

Lemony Chickpea Pasta with Peas

There are so many amazing pasta options nowadays; in addition to the traditional wheat, you can get pasta made from rice, quinoa, cauliflower, chickpeas, and more. I really like the chickpea variety; it's high-protein and gluten-free, and tastes so good. Here, I combine it with scallions, garlic, lemon, thyme, and peas for an easy, light, refreshing dish that won't leave you feeling lethargic the way wheat pasta sometimes can. Use the full amount of lemon juice and zest because they really pull the whole recipe together. If chickpea pasta isn't to your liking, you can sub any type of pasta.

Cook the pasta according to the package directions.

Meanwhile, in a large skillet, heat 2 tablespoons of the oil over medium-low heat. Add the garlic, thyme, and lemon zest and cook, stirring occasionally, until the garlic is golden, but not browned, 4 to 5 minutes.

Drain the pasta, reserving 1 cup of the water, and add the pasta to the skillet, along with the lemon juice, peas, scallions, salt, pepper, pasta water, and the remaining tablespoon of oil. Heat, tossing to combine, until warmed through, 3 to 4 minutes. Serve sprinkled with the Parmesan, if using.

Seven-Vegetable and Herb Soup

You may think you know vegetable soup—but wait until you try this. This is one of the healthiest, most antioxidant-rich, and delicious soups I've ever created. Just take a look at the ingredient list bursting with simple and readily accessible superfoods, and you'll already feel better! Crusty bread is a wonderful accompaniment.

In a medium pot, heat the oil over medium-high heat. Add the onion, carrots, and celery and cook, stirring occasionally, until the onion is softened, but not browned, about 5 minutes. Add the garlic and cook, stirring, for about a minute more.

Add the broth, water, potatoes, thyme, and salt and bring to a boil, then reduce the heat and simmer, partially covered, for 15 minutes.

Add the tomatoes, green beans, and broccoli and simmer until the vegetables are tender, 5 to 10 minutes. Adjust the salt according to taste. Divide into individual bowls, garnish with the basil, and serve.

2 tablespoons olive oil
1 large yellow onion, diced
2 carrots, peeled and diced
2 stalks celery, diced
3 cloves garlic, minced
1 quart plus 1½ cups low-sodium vegetable broth
1 cup water
3 (½-pound) unpeeled Yukon gold potatoes, cut into 1-inch chunks
1 tablespoon fresh thyme leaves
½ teaspoon sea salt
2 cups (about 3 whole) diced tomatoes
¼ pound green beans, cut into 1-inch pieces
1 cup small broccoli florets
⅓ cup minced fresh basil

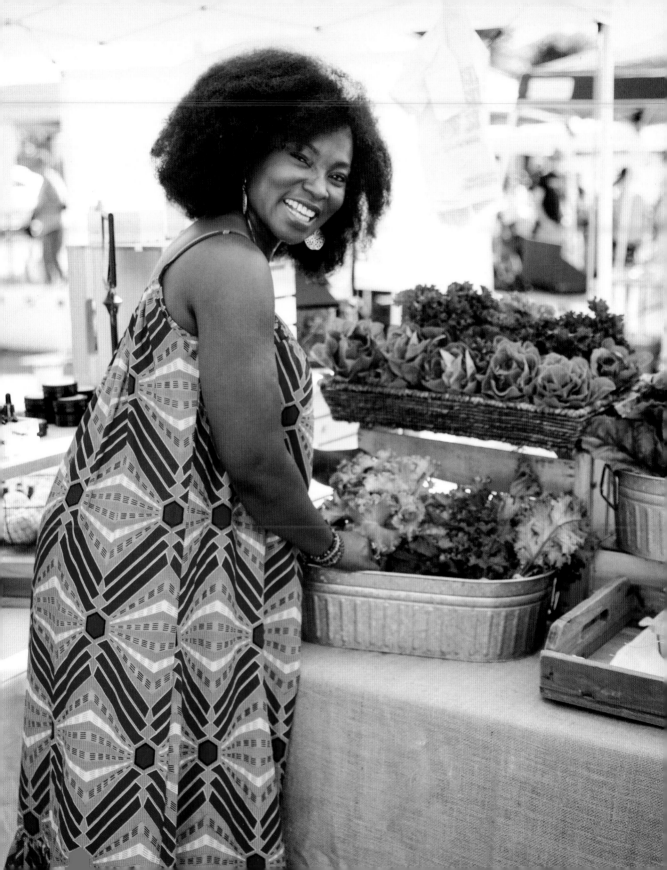

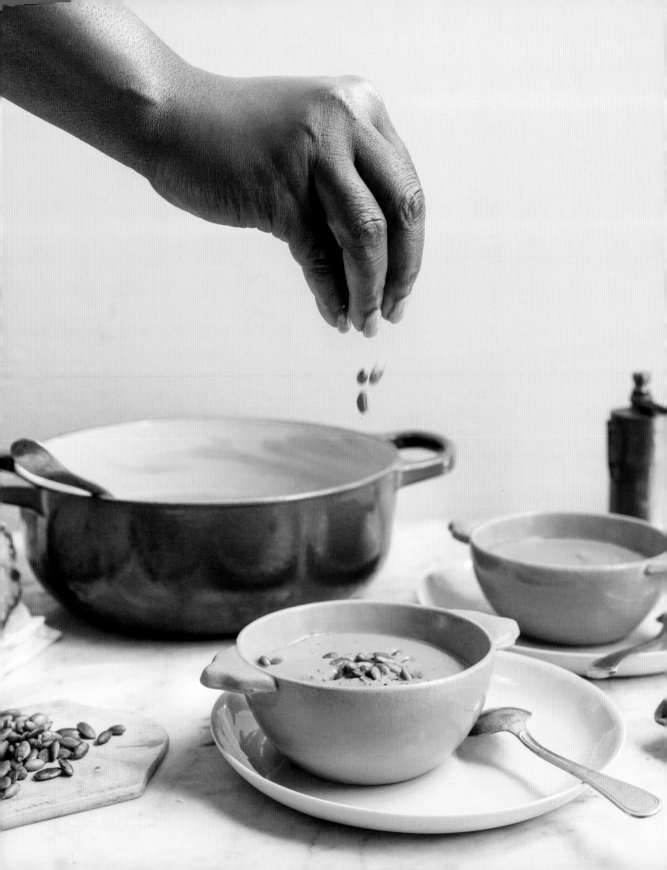

Butternut Squash Soup

GF, DF

SERVES 6

3 tablespoons olive oil
3¼ pounds butternut
squash, peeled,
seeded, and cut into
2-inch cubes
1 large onion, chopped
4 cloves garlic,
chopped
3 scallions, chopped
4 cups low-sodium
vegetable or chicken
broth, plus more if
needed
½ teaspoon sea salt
¼ teaspoon freshly
ground black pepper

In 2003, my family and a few of our friends spent an incredible week in Jamaica at the sweet little Endless Summer Villa. The first night, the appetizer was a bowl of the most exquisitely delicious butternut squash soup any of us had ever tasted. In fact, it was so good, everyone asked for it again the next day for lunch. The soup was so creamy, it felt like dreamy clouds in your mouth even though it had zero dairy. I wanted the recipe badly. The day we were leaving, I asked the chef for it. I can still hear his boisterous laugh. "Sis!" he said. "Nobody has recipe, man. We cook only." I laughed right back and told him I could relate: "We Africans cook with our eyes and heart, too," I said. "Just tell me all the ingredients you used, and I will figure out the rest." He kindly obliged, and when I got home, I tested batch after batch, finally coming up with a very close approximation. It's my favorite soup and, rather than make you guess my recipe, here it is for you to enjoy.

You do not want to rush the process as you caramelize the squash, onion, garlic, and scallions; it is the secret sauce here and brings the natural sweetness of this soup. Oh goodness, the depth and richness of it blows my mind every time, and I have been cooking and eating this soup for more than nineteen years.

It's also really good topped with crumbled Plantain Tapé (page 255), toasted pepitas, or sautéed greens or, of course, eaten with a good piece of crusty bread.

In a large pot, heat the oil over medium heat. Add the squash, onion, garlic, and scallions and cook, stirring occasionally, until the ingredients start to caramelize, 7 to 10 minutes. (Don't rush this step; it's important for the flavor of the soup.)

Stir in the broth, salt, and pepper and bring to a boil over high heat. Reduce the heat and simmer, covered, until the squash is tender, 20 to 30 minutes. Let cool slightly, then blend in a blender until creamy, working in batches, if necessary. If the soup is too thick, add a little more broth, but it shouldn't be runny. Season to taste with a little more salt and pepper, and serve.

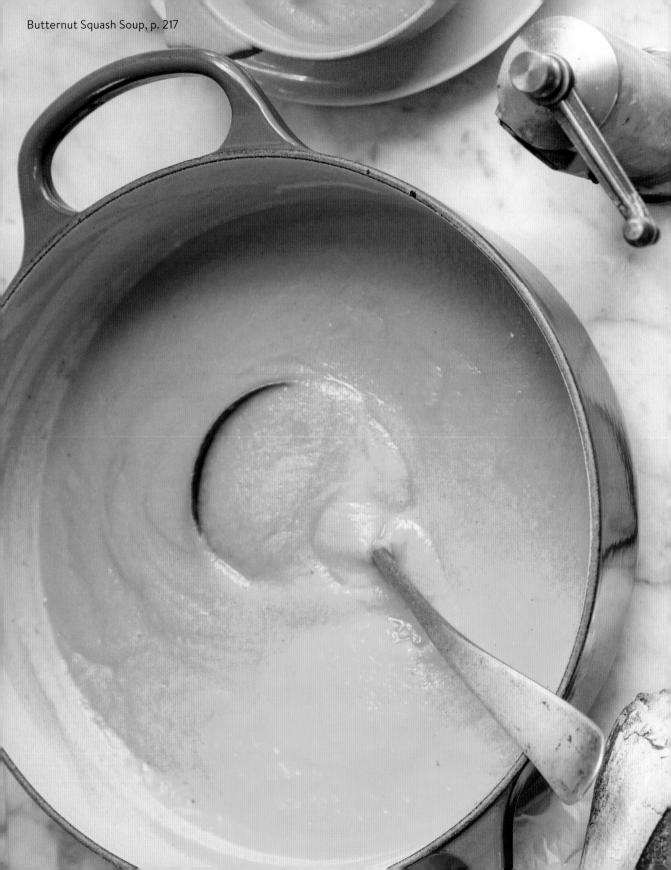
Butternut Squash Soup, p. 217

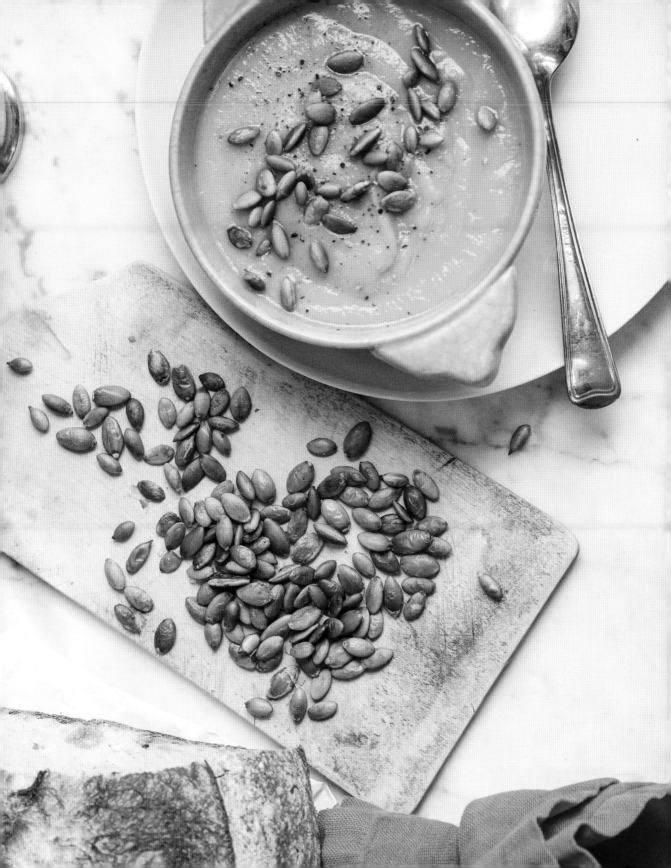

Lentil Stew

3 tablespoons olive oil
1 onion, diced
4 stalks celery, diced
3 carrots, peeled, diced
2 cloves garlic, minced
2 cups brown lentils, picked over and rinsed
1 teaspoon ground cumin
1 teaspoon grated peeled fresh ginger
1 teaspoon dried oregano
1 teaspoon smoked paprika
6 cups low-sodium chicken or vegetable broth
10 ounces frozen spinach, thawed
⅓ cup chopped dried cranberries
Sea salt
Freshly ground pepper

This rustic lentil stew will leave you feeling warm and toasty while providing valuable health benefits—perfect for colder weather. The delightfully fragrant spices—ginger, cumin, and oregano—are anti-inflammatories and help promote good digestion. Meanwhile, the mighty lentils are rich in fiber, folate, and potassium, making them a great choice for the heart and for managing blood pressure and cholesterol. They are also a source of energizing iron and vitamin B_1, which helps maintain a steady heartbeat. The dish is vegan if you use vegetable broth. You can also use fresh spinach when it's in season and cheaper.

In a medium pot, heat the oil over medium heat. Add the onion and cook, stirring occasionally, until translucent, about 5 minutes. Add the celery, carrots, and garlic and cook, stirring occasionally, until just glistening, about 5 minutes.

Stir in the lentils, cumin, ginger, oregano, and smoked paprika, followed by the broth. Cover and bring to a boil over medium-high heat, then reduce the heat and simmer until the lentils are tender, about 30 minutes, adding water if needed.

Stir in the spinach and cranberries, season with salt and pepper, and cook for about 15 minutes more.

Serve with rice or crusty bread.

1/4 cup olive oil
1 large onion, diced
3 cloves garlic, minced
4 tomatoes (1 pound), finely diced
3 scallions, thinly sliced
1/2 teaspoon crushed red pepper flakes (optional)
1/2 teaspoon grated peeled fresh ginger
2 carrots, peeled, halved lengthwise and cut into 1-inch chunks
1 yellow bell pepper, seeded and cut into 1-inch-thick slices
1 teaspoon Bragg Liquid Aminos or coconut aminos
1/2 teaspoon sea salt
1 pound green beans, cut into 1-inch pieces
1 zucchini, quartered lengthwise and cut into 1-inch chunks

Farmer's Harvest Vegetable Stew

I love fresh-tomato-based anything, and this stew is no exception. Did you know tomato is one fruit (yes, it is technically a fruit, though I won't add it to my fruit salad) that benefits the entire body? It turns out tomatoes are good for our skin, eyes, heart (thanks to the abundance of lycopene), and gut health (thanks to the fluid and fiber content). Tomatoes are also high in vitamins including vitamin C, which is good for overall immune-system health, and vitamin K, which is good for bone health. I am such a visual eater, and tomatoes make everything look pretty and taste even better. With onions, which I personally believe bring the best out of tomatoes, and a hint of ginger, this dish is a real mouth pleaser. As with most of my dishes, the goal is that you not only make it but make it yours—use your favorite herbs and vegetables, and have fun with it. Serve with Nutty Spiced Rice (page 245), Quinoa with Cilantro and Lemon (page 242), or, if you really want to make it an all-vegetable meal, Stir-Fried Cauliflower Rice (page 241).

In a large skillet, heat the oil over medium heat. Add the onion and cook, stirring frequently, until translucent, about 5 minutes. Add the garlic and cook, stirring, for about 1 minute.

Add the tomatoes, scallions, red pepper flakes, if using, and ginger and cook, stirring occasionally, until the tomatoes begin to soften, about 7 minutes. Add the carrots, bell pepper, aminos, and salt and cook, stirring occasionally, for about 5 minutes, taste and adjust the seasoning as needed. Add the green beans and zucchini, mix well, and simmer, covered, until the vegetables are crisp-tender, about 5 minutes. Cook longer if your family enjoys a softer texture, then serve.

SERVES 4 TO 6

Black Bean and Corn Stew

Growing up, I watched Mami soak beans in cold water overnight before cooking them, a method used for centuries by Indigenous populations all over the world. Mami may not have known the biochemical reasons it was beneficial, but she almost surely understood that it helped them cook more evenly and quickly and minimized their gassy effect.

This is a popular bean dish in Cameroon and in other West African countries because of its deliciousness. The Cameroonian name for this dish is cornchaff; it is usually made with dried corn. I made a few changes to adapt it to my American culture, and I now love it even more. This dish is a party in your mouth—think ginger, garlic, leeks, cumin, and the sweetness of corn and bell pepper, all doing a merry dance. This dish is usually a meal on its own, but as the proclaimed queen of stretching meals, I like to serve it with Plantain Tapé (page 255). You can also create a lovely bowl with Kale Salad (page 249). Add some avocado with a splash of lemon and have another meal, or add a soft-boiled egg or spread the stew on a slice of toast for breakfast—the options are endless.

In a medium pot, combine the beans and cold water. Bring to a boil over high heat, then reduce the heat and simmer until tender, 45 to 60 minutes, adding more water as needed. Drain and rinse the beans, then set aside.

In a medium pot, heat the oil over medium heat. Add the onion, leeks, and bay leaf and cook, stirring occasionally, until the onion is translucent, about 5 minutes. Add the garlic and cumin and cook, stirring, for 30 seconds. Add the tomatoes and cook, stirring occasionally, for 10 minutes.

Add the scallions, bell pepper, ginger, Scotch bonnet pepper or habanero, if using, and salt and cook, stirring occasionally, for 4 minutes. Stir in 3 cups of the beans, the corn, broth, and Better Than Bouillon or coconut aminos. Reduce the heat and simmer for 20 minutes or until thickened. Remove the bay leaf and add more salt, if needed. Serve.

2 cups dried black beans, picked over and soaked overnight in cold water, then drained and rinsed (will make extra beans for storing)
6 cups cold water, plus more as needed
⅓ cup olive oil
1 onion, finely chopped
⅓ cup diced leeks, pale green and white parts
1 bay leaf
3 cloves garlic, minced
1 teaspoon ground cumin
1 pound tomatoes, diced
3 scallions, finely chopped
1 yellow bell pepper, seeded and diced
1 teaspoon grated peeled fresh ginger
1 Scotch bonnet pepper or habanero (optional)
½ teaspoon sea salt
2 cups fresh or frozen corn kernels, thawed
1 cup low-sodium vegetable broth
1 teaspoon Better Than Bouillon or coconut aminos

NOTE: Cooking dried beans saves time and money. The 2 cups of dry beans this recipe calls for will give you enough for this dish plus the Black Bean Burgers (page 210). You can freeze any unused cooked beans for when you want to make this dish again.

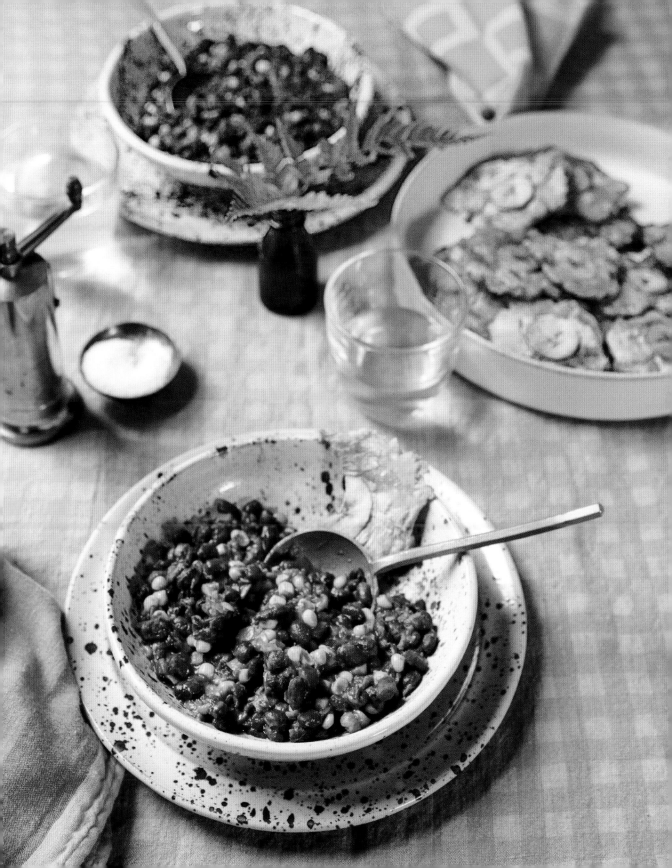

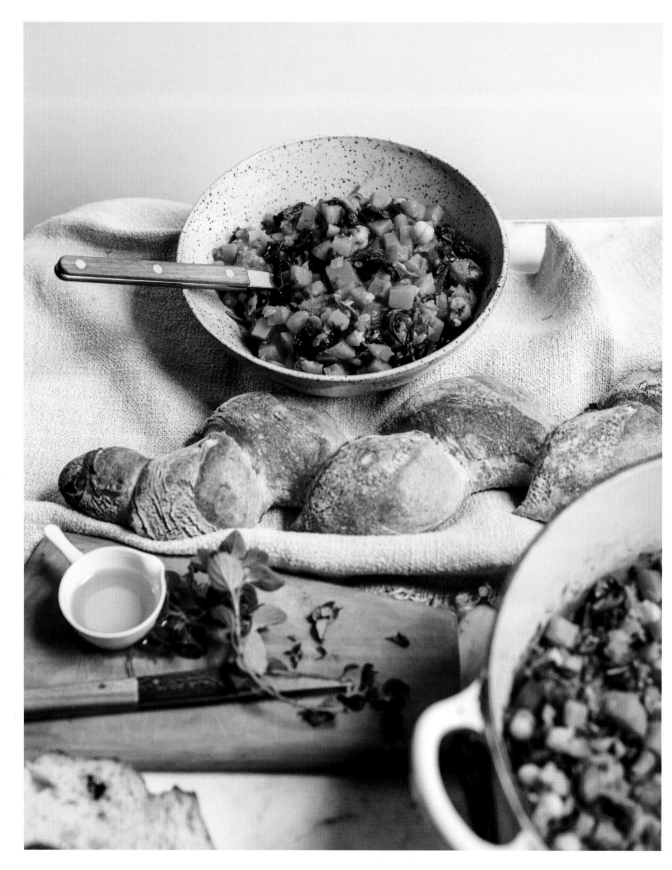

Soufico

MEDITERRANEAN VEGETABLE STEW

Soufico is a traditional dish from Greece and a particularly popular meal on Ikaria. This island in the Aegean, about forty miles off the eastern coast of Turkey, is reportedly one of the healthiest regions in the world, boasting a large population of centenarians who still lead active lives. I discovered this delicious and healthy dish through American National Geographic fellow and *New York Times* best-selling author Dan Buettner. Let's all dig into the fountain of youth, shall we? Serve over a bowl of farro, rice, fonio, or whatever you are loving at the moment. You can't go wrong with this stew.

2 tablespoons olive oil
1 red onion, roughly chopped
3 cloves garlic, minced
2 cups chopped juicy tomatoes
2 large carrots, peeled and cut into ½-inch dice
1 large sweet potato (about 1 pound), peeled and cut into ½-inch dice
½ teaspoon sea salt
¼ teaspoon freshly ground black pepper
3 cups vegetable broth
1½ cups cooked chickpeas
1 yellow bell pepper, seeded and cut into ½-inch dice
1 tablespoon chopped fresh oregano
1 teaspoon chopped fresh thyme leaves
2 bay leaves, preferably fresh
6 ounces baby spinach
½ cup finely chopped fresh flat-leaf parsley
Extra-virgin olive oil, for garnish
8 large fresh basil leaves, chopped

In a large Dutch oven or other heavy pot, heat the olive oil over medium heat until shimmering, but not smoking. Add the onion and cook until translucent, stirring occasionally, about 3 minutes. Add the garlic and cook, stirring, for 1 minute more.

Add the tomatoes and cook, stirring often, for about 5 minutes. Add the carrots, sweet potato, salt, and pepper and continue cooking, stirring occasionally, for about 5 minutes more.

Add the broth, chickpeas, bell pepper, oregano, thyme, and bay leaves. Bring to a boil over high heat, reduce the heat to low, and cook, covered and stirring occasionally, until the sweet potato and carrots are tender and the liquid is thickened, 20 to 25 minutes.

Stir in the spinach and cook for 2 minutes more, then stir in the parsley. Remove from the heat and discard the bay leaves. Finish with a generous drizzle of extra-virgin olive oil and the basil and serve.

Chana Masala

CHICKPEA CURRY

I love traditional tomato-based Indian curries, and this one is no exception. It's so tasty, and in addition to green beans, chickpeas, and tomatoes, it contains spinach, dates, and red pepper flakes. Plus, it is high in protein and fiber, which are good for satiety and gut health. Serve with plantains, rice, roti, or naan.

In a medium skillet, heat the oil over medium-high heat. Add the onion and cook, stirring occasionally, until translucent, about 5 minutes. Add the garlic and cook, stirring, for 1 minute.

Add the green beans and ginger and continue cooking, stirring occasionally, for about 5 minutes, adding a little water or broth to prevent sticking, if needed. Stir in the chickpeas, tomatoes, curry powder, cumin, red pepper flakes, dates, and remaining liquid and cook until thickened and the flavors blend together, about 15 minutes more.

Stir in the spinach and cook for about 2 minutes (don't overcook it), then stir in the parsley, lemon juice, and salt and black pepper to taste.

Serve.

¼ cup olive oil

1 cup finely chopped onion

3 large cloves garlic, minced

6 ounces green beans, cut into 1-inch pieces

1 tablespoon grated peeled fresh ginger

1½ cups water or low-sodium vegetable broth

3 cups cooked chickpeas

2 cups roughly chopped tomatoes

1 tablespoon curry powder

1 teaspoon ground cumin

½ teaspoon crushed red pepper flakes

1 Medjool date, pitted and chopped

2 packed cups baby spinach, chopped

2 tablespoons chopped fresh flat-leaf parsley

1 tablespoon fresh lemon juice

Sea salt

Freshly ground black pepper

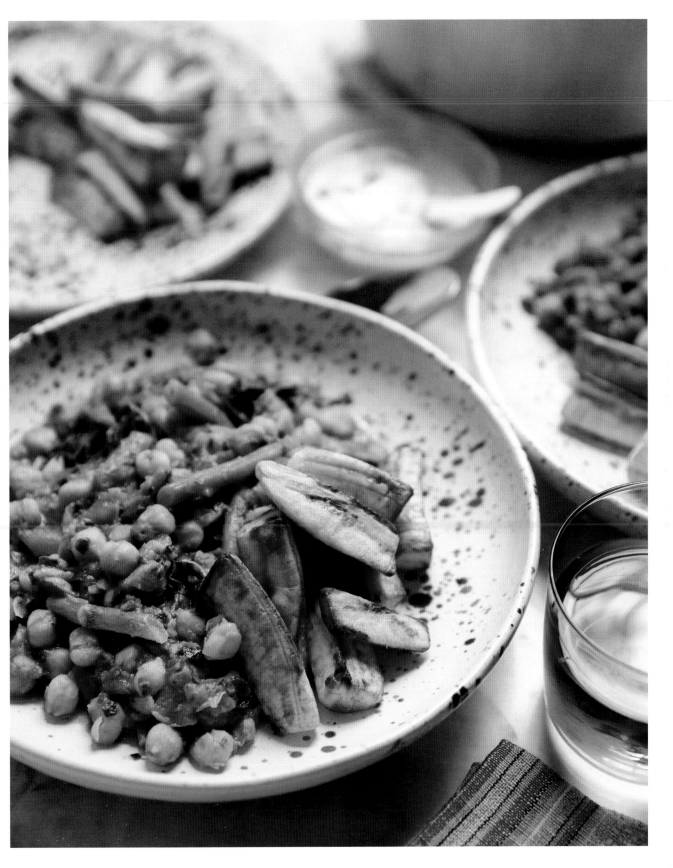

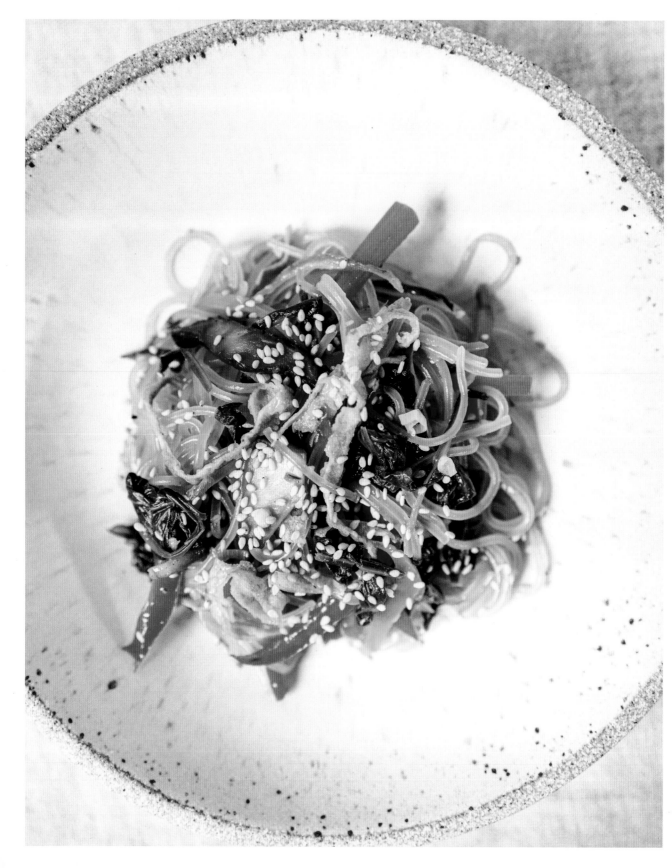

GF, DF

SERVES 4 TO 6

Japchae

KOREAN SWEET POTATO NOODLES AND VEGETABLES

Don't let the length of this classic Korean recipe fool you—there's a fair amount of prep, but it's all very straightforward, and once you start cooking, it goes quickly. Plus, the result is so delightful and packed with nutrients. For instance, shiitake mushrooms, just one of the many amazing ingredients in this dish, have really high amounts of natural copper, a mineral that supports healthy blood vessels, bones, and the immune system.

For the egg garnish, if using, in a small bowl, whisk together the egg and salt. Heat a small skillet over medium heat. Add the olive oil and swirl the pan so it covers the bottom. Add the egg and tilt the pan to create a thin layer of egg. Let it cook for about a minute, then flip it over, turn off the heat, and let it sit for 1 minute more. When cool, slice into thin strips and set aside.

Fill a large bowl with ice water and bring a large pot of water to a boil. Add the spinach to the boiling water and blanch for about 30 seconds. Remove with a strainer, keeping the water boiling for the noodles, and immediately immerse the spinach in the ice water until cold to stop the cooking process.

Drain the spinach, squeeze to remove any excess water, and roughly chop it. Transfer to a large bowl, toss with 1 teaspoon each of the tamari and sesame oil, and set aside.

Stir the noodles into the boiling water and cook, stirring occasionally, until soft and chewy, about 6 minutes. Drain and rinse under cold running water, then cut the noodles using a pair of kitchen scissors into about 6-inch lengths. Place in the bowl next to the spinach and toss with 2 teaspoons of the sesame oil, 2 teaspoons of the tamari, and 2 teaspoons of the honey.

In a large skillet, heat 2 teaspoons of olive oil over medium-high heat. Add the onion, scallions, and a pinch of salt and cook, stirring

EGG GARNISH (OPTIONAL)

1 large egg
Pinch sea salt
1 teaspoon olive oil

NOODLES

6 ounces baby spinach
2 tablespoons tamari, divided
2 tablespoons toasted sesame oil, divided
8 ounces sweet potato noodles (dangmyeon)
1 tablespoon plus 2 teaspoons raw honey, divided (see Note)
1 tablespoon plus 2 teaspoons olive oil, divided
1 onion, thinly sliced
3 scallions, cut into 1-inch pieces
Sea salt
2 cloves garlic, minced
4 button mushrooms, sliced
4 shiitake mushrooms, sliced
1 carrot, julienned
½ red bell pepper, seeded and thinly sliced
½ yellow bell pepper, seeded and thinly sliced
½ teaspoon freshly ground black pepper
1 tablespoon toasted sesame seeds
½ teaspoon crushed red pepper flakes (optional)

(Continued)

occasionally, for about 2 minutes. Add the garlic and cook, stirring occasionally, for 1 minute, then transfer the onion mixture to the noodle bowl, reserving the skillet.

Heat 2 teaspoons of olive oil in the skillet over medium-high heat. Add the mushrooms and let cook for 2 minutes without moving, then flip, add a pinch of salt, and cook until tender and lightly browned, about 3 minutes more. Transfer to the noodle bowl, reserving the skillet.

Heat 1 teaspoon of olive oil in the skillet over medium-high heat. Add the carrots and cook, stirring often, for 30 seconds. Add the bell peppers and cook, stirring often, for 20 seconds more. Transfer to the noodle bowl.

Add the remaining 1 tablespoon of tamari, 1 tablespoon of honey, 1 tablespoon of sesame oil, and the black pepper to the noodle bowl. Mix all the ingredients by hand until completely combined and check the seasonings. Add the egg garnish, if using, sesame seeds, and red pepper flakes, if using, and toss again. Transfer to a large plate and serve at room temperature.

NOTE: Do not serve honey to babies twelve months or younger, as it may cause infant botulism. Use maple syrup instead.

Sweet Potato Black Bean Stew

2 tablespoons olive oil
1 large onion, chopped
4 cloves garlic, minced
2 scallions, thinly
  sliced
2 teaspoons ground
  cumin
¼ teaspoon sea salt,
  or to taste
1 pound roma
  tomatoes, chopped,
  or 1 (14½-ounce) can
  crushed tomatoes
1 medium sweet
  potato, peeled and
  diced
2½ cups low-sodium
  vegetable broth
3 cups cooked black
  beans, drained;
  if using canned,
  drained and rinsed
½ teaspoon crushed
  red pepper flakes
  (optional)
Juice of ½ lime

My mother first made this for my youngest child when he was about nine months old. She used adzuki beans because they are easier for a baby to digest than black beans. I loved the dish so much I made a grownup version using black beans, and it's been on rotation at our home ever since. Enjoy it with rice or roasted plantains and salad.

In a large pot, heat the oil over medium-high heat. Add the onion and cook, stirring occasionally, until fragrant and softened, about 4 minutes. Add the garlic, scallions, cumin, and salt and cook, stirring, for about 30 seconds. Add the tomatoes, mix well, and cook until the liquid is almost gone, about 10 minutes, stirring every few minutes to make sure the mixture is not sticking to the pan.

Add the sweet potatoes and cook, stirring occasionally, for about 1 minute. Add the broth and bring to a gentle boil, then cover, reduce the heat, and simmer until the sweet potatoes are fork-tender, 12 to 14 minutes.

Stir in the beans, red pepper flakes, if using, and lime juice and bring to a boil. Adjust the seasoning to taste. Reduce the heat to a simmer and continue cooking until thickened, about 7 minutes more. Serve.

Did you know that for centuries, cumin has been used for medicinal purposes? My mami would say it is good for digestion, and now I am seeing the science that backs that up. Cumin is also very dense in iron, providing almost 20 percent of your daily iron requirement in one teaspoon.

6 large bell peppers,
  any color
2 tablespoons olive
  oil, plus more for the
  baking dish
½ cup diced sweet
  onions
1 cup sliced shiitake
  mushrooms
Sea salt
Freshly ground black
  pepper
2 cloves garlic, minced
1½ cups cooked black
  beans, drained;
  if using canned,
  drained and rinsed
1½ cups cooked brown
  rice
1 cup fresh or thawed
  frozen corn kernels
1 cup diced tomatoes
2 scallions, thinly
  sliced
1 teaspoon Bragg
  Liquid Aminos, or to
  taste
½ teaspoon ground
  cumin
½ teaspoon Italian
  seasoning
½ teaspoon smoked
  paprika
1 cup shredded
  mozzarella cheese,
  divided (optional)

Stuffed Bell Peppers

This is a popular meatless Monday dish in my house because it tastes great and looks beautiful. Of course, I also like it because it's good for you. Bell peppers are nutrient-dense, high in vitamin C, and contain more than thirty types of carotenoids, which researchers have found can help heal eyes and ward off eye disease.

There truly is nothing I haven't either at the very least tried or stuffed into bell peppers, especially when trying to makeover a particularly large batch of leftovers at home. Don't stop with this recipe, next time try adding some ground meat or cooked lentils or quinoa to change things up a little—or a lot.

Preheat the oven to 350°F. Lightly coat an 11 × 7-inch glass or ceramic baking dish with oil.

Cut off the tops of the peppers. Chop the flesh from the tops and set aside. Scoop the seeds and white membrane from the insides of the peppers and discard, then place the peppers onto the prepared baking dish and set aside.

In a medium skillet, heat the oil over medium heat. Add the onions and cook, stirring occasionally, until translucent, about 4 minutes. Add the mushrooms and season with salt and pepper and cook, stirring often, for 1 minute. Add the garlic and cook, stirring, for 30 seconds.

Transfer the mixture to a large mixing bowl. Add the beans, rice, corn, tomatoes, scallions, reserved chopped pepper tops, aminos, cumin, Italian seasoning, smoked paprika, and salt and pepper to taste, and mix well, then stir in ½ cup of the cheese, if using.

Stuff the peppers tightly with the filling and top each with some of the remaining ½ cup of cheese, if using. Cover with foil (at home I cover first with parchment paper and then with foil to hold it in place) and bake for 20 minutes. Uncover and bake until the cheese is melted and browned and the peppers are tender, about 10 minutes more. Serve.

NOTE: I love my food colorful and vibrant. I use red, yellow, orange, and green peppers. You can go with your pepper of choice or join my multicolor train. They can be made vegan by removing the cheese; they are also easy to make in advance and bake or reheat later.

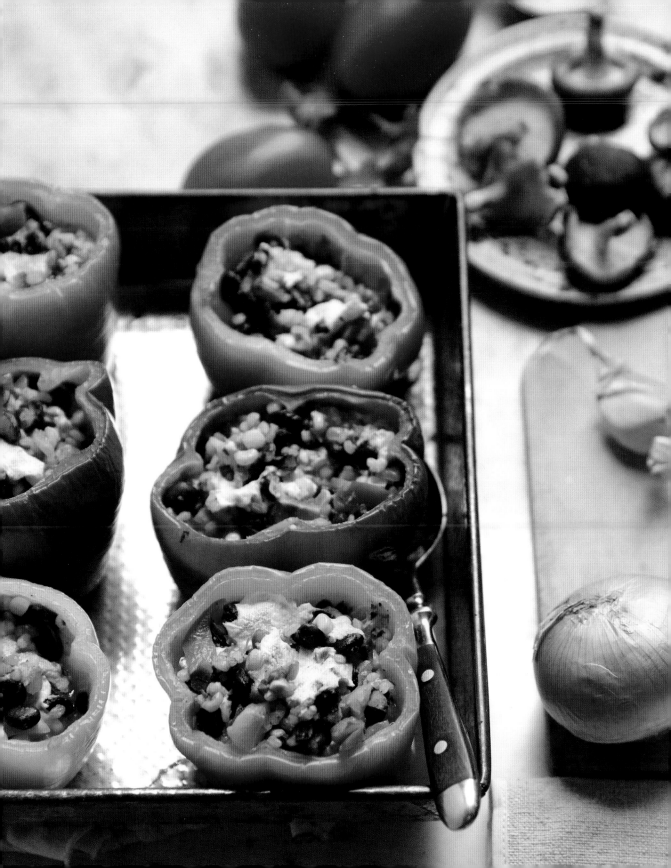

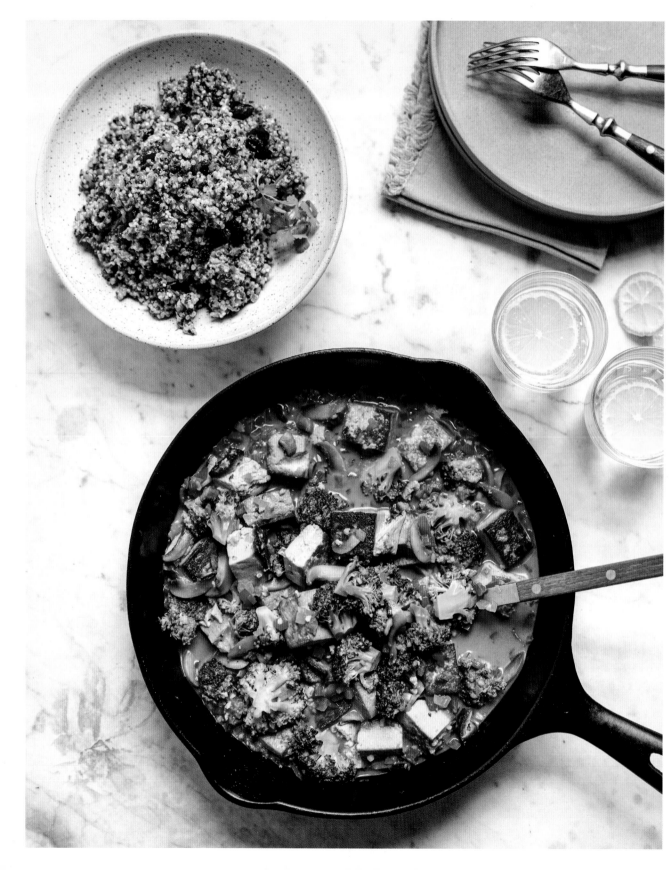

2 (14-ounce) packages firm tofu, drained, pressed (see sidebar, page 86), and cut into 1-inch cubes
½ cup tamari
¼ cup olive oil, divided
½ cup chopped onions
½ pound shiitake mushrooms, sliced
2 cups low-sodium broth
3 tablespoons raw honey (see Note)
1 tablespoon Dijon mustard
1 teaspoon grated peeled fresh ginger
3 cloves garlic, minced
½ red bell pepper, cut into ½-inch dice
2 broccoli crowns (1 pound), cut into florets

Tofu and Mushrooms Stir-Fry

I love my food to look pretty, taste good, and be healthy, and this dish checks all the boxes. This stir-fry combines two superfoods, tofu and mushrooms. Tofu is a good source of complete protein and has an abundance of several anti-inflammatory, antioxidant, and phytochemical properties; mushrooms are high in vitamin B. The umami flavor of the tamari and hint of honey give this dish such a rich flavor, and the mushroom adds a smoky depth. I have found that even the pickiest eaters who won't eat their forbidden broccoli will venture to suck the velvety sauce off it. Listen, don't skip the tofu press if you can; it makes a huge difference. This is another versatile recipe that you can play with and make your own—swap zucchini for broccoli or oyster mushrooms for the tofu, for example. This dish will bring out your inner Julia Child. Serve over Quinoa with Cilantro and Lemon (page 242) or Stir-Fried Cauliflower Rice (page 241) or your favorite noodles.

In a shallow dish, marinate the tofu in the tamari for at east 2 hours, or overnight, covered in the refrigerator, turning occasionally.

Remove the tofu from the marinade, reserving the liquid. In a large skillet, heat 3 tablespoons of the oil over medium heat. Add the tofu and brown on two sides, 3 to 4 minutes. Transfer to a plate, reserving the pan.

Add the remaining tablespoon of oil to the pan and heat over medium heat. Add the onions and mushrooms and cook, stirring occasionally, until the onions are soft, about 5 minutes.

Meanwhile, in a medium bowl, stir together the broth, honey, mustard, ginger, garlic, and bell pepper. When the onions are soft, add the mixture to the pan and stir to combine. Add the tofu and reserved marinade and simmer over medium heat for 1 minute.

Add the broccoli and simmer, stirring occasionally, for 3 minutes more. Remove from the heat and let sit for 5 minutes before serving.

NOTE: Do not serve raw honey to babies twelve months or younger, as it may cause infant botulism. Use maple syrup instead.

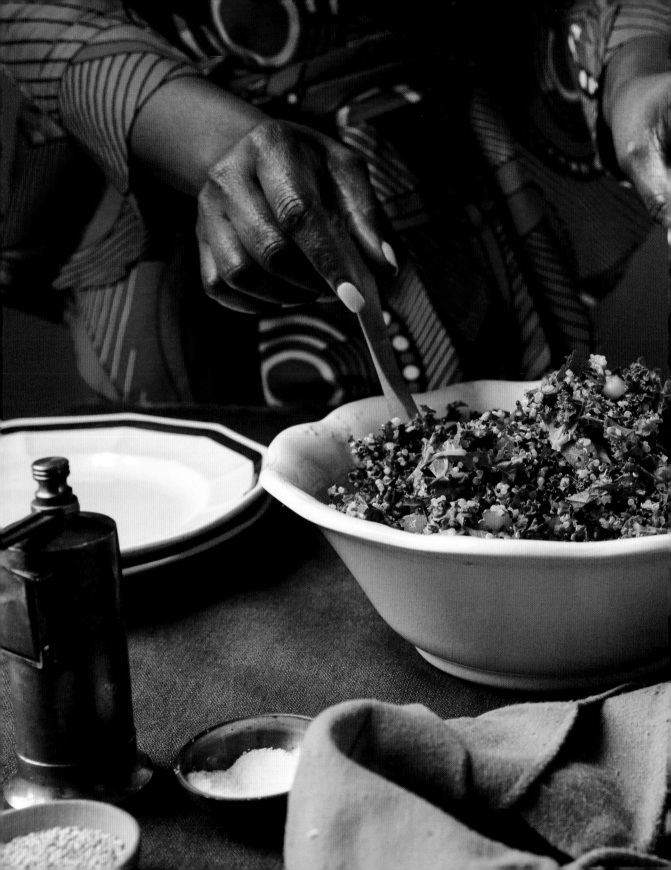

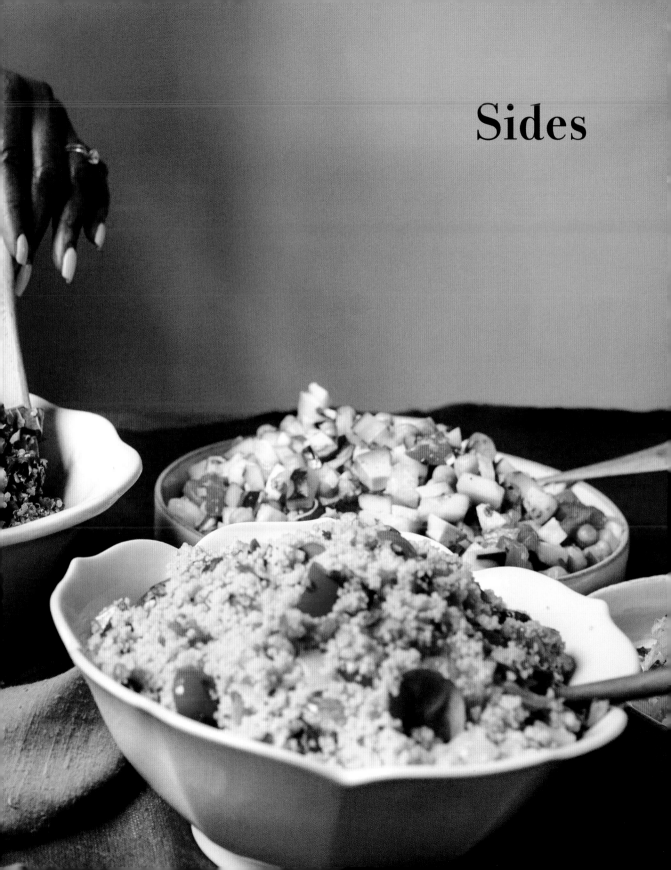

Sides

Side dishes are, in my opinion, very underrated and are usually somewhat of an afterthought, but never underestimate the power of an amazing side dish. It can be the glue that holds dinner together and, when money is a little tight, can stretch your main dish like an elastic band. Sides are also a great way to get more vegetables, fruits, and grains into your diet and boost the nutritional value of your meal. Of course, choosing the right side dish makes all the difference, and it should always complement the entrée. Here are some of my most popular and versatile sides. A far cry from classic steamed veggies and green salads, they combine a variety of flavors and textures, look as good as they taste, and are super healthy.

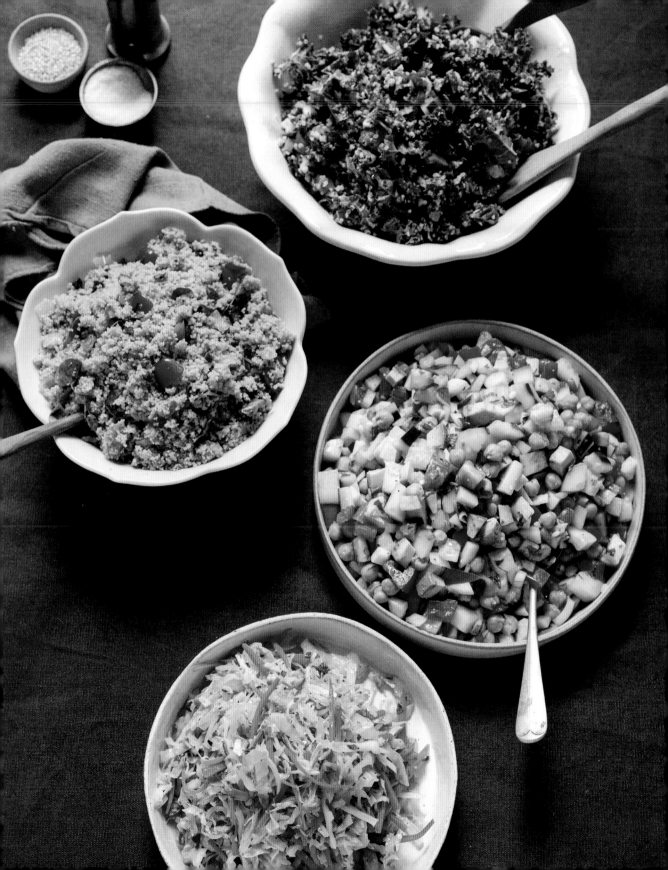

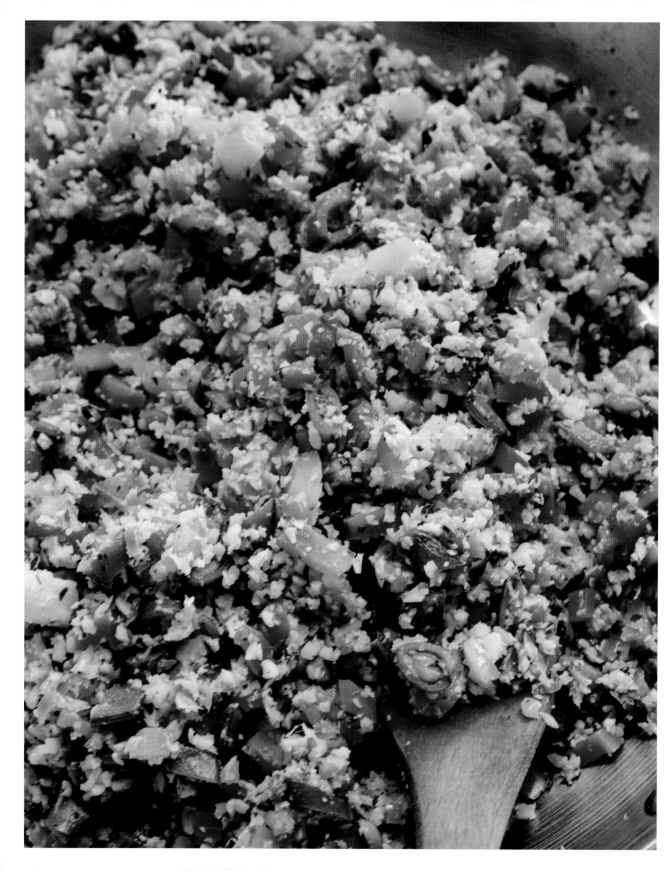

1 medium head cauliflower, separated into florets or 2½ cups cauliflower rice
3 tablespoons olive oil
1 small red onion, diced
1 clove garlic, minced
2 small carrots, diced
1 red bell pepper, seeded and diced
1 yellow bell pepper, seeded and diced
2 cups diced sugar snap peas
2 scallions, thinly sliced
2 tablespoons chopped fresh basil
2 tablespoons chopped fresh flat-leaf parsley
1 teaspoon sesame oil
½ teaspoon crushed red pepper flakes
1 to 2 tablespoons coconut aminos
Sea salt
Freshly ground black pepper

Stir-Fried Cauliflower Rice

If there is one family of food that is best at improving gut health and thus the immune system it is the cruciferous vegetables, which includes the humble cauliflower. White foods get a bad rap, but cauliflower is super nutritious and very versatile. I love it in rice form, particularly when it's stir-fried like this with other vegetables. You can easily turn this side into a complete meal by adding some form of protein. If you aren't a fan of cauliflower rice, this recipe will make you a believer, and if you already love cauliflower rice, you will love this even more. It is bold, screaming loudly, "Dig in!" Bell peppers and sugar snap peas add not only sweetness to the dish but also a pop of color. The hint of toasted sesame oil takes it to another level. Serve warm with Chana Masala (page 226), Grandma's Meatballs (page 140), Herb- and Parmesan-Crusted Chicken (page 173), or Lemony Salmon Kebabs (page 198).

If starting with cauliflower florets, place them in a food processor and pulse just until they resemble rice. (If you do not have a food processor, you can use a hand grater or knife.)

Heat a large skillet or wok over medium heat. Add the olive oil and onion and cook, stirring occasionally, until the onion is translucent, about 4 minutes. Add the garlic and carrots and cook, stirring occasionally, for 2 minutes. Add the bell peppers and cook until almost tender, about 3 minutes then add the sugar snap peas and cook for about 2 minutes more, stirring occasionally.

Add the cauliflower rice, scallions, basil, parsley, sesame oil, red pepper flakes, and coconut aminos to taste. Stir until the cauliflower rice is tender, about 3 minutes. Season with a little salt and black pepper to taste and serve.

NOTE: Cut everything about the same size for even cooking.

2 tablespoons olive oil
1 small red onion, finely diced
1 clove garlic, minced
1 cup quinoa, rinsed
2 cups water or low-sodium broth of your choice
⅓ cup dried cranberries
½ teaspoon sea salt, or to taste
Zest and juice of 1 lemon
⅓ cup chopped fresh cilantro
Freshly ground black pepper

Quinoa with Cilantro and Lemon

Hundreds of years ago, the Inca people considered quinoa a sacred food. Today, this ancient grain's popularity has grown exponentially as the demand for nutritious, gluten-free grain alternatives has soared. Quinoa is a nutritional powerhouse, loaded with fiber, protein, iron, folate, and magnesium. Adding fresh lemon juice doesn't only add flavor; its high vitamin C content makes it easier for the body to absorb the plant-based iron that quinoa is loved for. This is especially important for those with an iron deficiency who don't eat meat. While you can serve the quinoa alongside whatever main dish you like, try it with Chana Masala (page 226) for a yummy meatless Monday dinner, Curried Chicken Stir-Fry (page 175), or Shrimp and Tomato Stew with Scallions (page 190).

In a large skillet, heat the oil over medium-high heat. Add the onion and cook, stirring occasionally, until translucent, about 4 minutes. Add the garlic and cook, stirring often, for 30 seconds, then add the quinoa and cook, stirring often, for 2 minutes more.

Stir in the water, cranberries, and salt. Bring to a boil, then reduce the heat to low, cover, and simmer for 20 minutes. Remove from the heat and let rest for 5 minutes without removing the lid. Fluff with a fork, add the lemon zest and juice and cilantro, and fluff again to incorporate. Season to taste with pepper and more salt, if needed. Serve.

NOTE: If you are new to the taste and world of quinoa, my recommendation is to cook it with your favorite broth instead of water; it lends so much more flavor to this ancient grain.

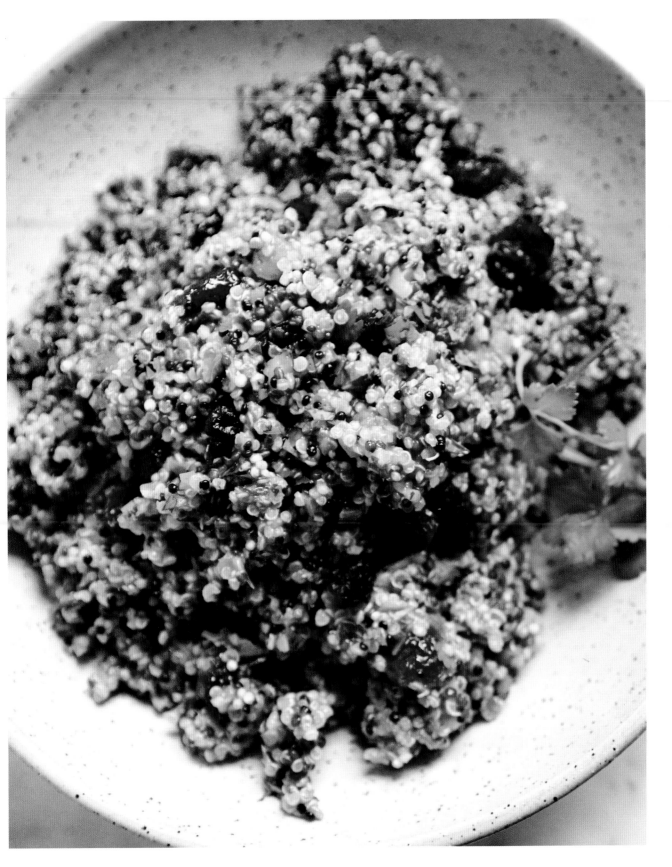

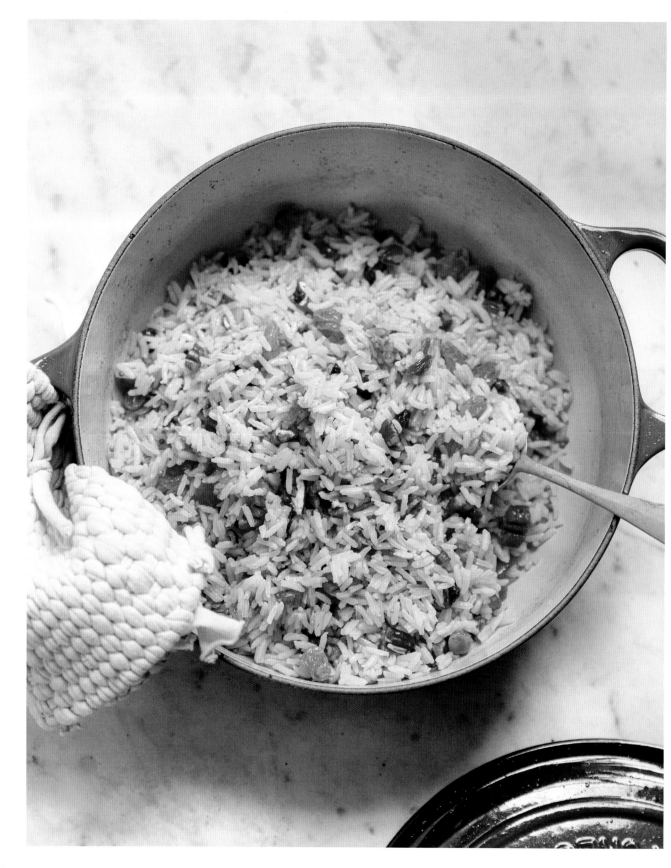

Nutty Spiced Rice

1½ cups basmati rice, rinsed until the water runs clear
2¼ cups water
10 whole cloves
3 bay leaves
2 cinnamon sticks
⅛ teaspoon ground turmeric
1 teaspoon sea salt
2 tablespoons olive oil
1 tablespoon butter or ghee
2 teaspoons mustard seeds
¼ cup chopped roasted pecans
¼ cup golden raisins

This is my all-time favorite side dish and a step up from your average rice pilaf. The nuts and spices combine for a warm, rich flavor that is incredible—and the health benefits are even better. Turmeric has long been known for its anti-inflammatory, antibacterial, and detoxifying properties, but recent studies have indicated that this spice can also be used to effectively treat Alzheimer's disease. The dish also has healthy fat from the nuts and healing benefits from the mustard seeds. Did you know that the mustard seeds have a history of use as a remedy in traditional medicine dating as far back as ancient Greek and Roman civilizations? Don't stop here—look for more ways to incorporate them into your diet. While you can pretty much pair this with any dish, I especially enjoy it with Maple-Glazed Chicken and Veggies (page 171), Shrimp and Tomato Stew with Scallions (page 190), Lemony Salmon Kebabs (page 198), and Tofu and Mushrooms Stir-Fry (page 235).

Place the rice in a medium saucepan with a lid. Add the water, cloves, bay leaves, cinnamon sticks, turmeric, and salt. Bring to a boil over high heat, then reduce the heat to low, cover, and cook for 15 minutes. Remove from the heat and let rest for 10 minutes without removing the lid.

Meanwhile, in a small skillet, heat the oil and butter over medium-high heat. Add the mustard seeds and stir until they start to pop, about 1 minute. Add the pecans and raisins and cook, stirring constantly, for 30 seconds.

Pour the mixture on top of the rice and fluff with a fork. Remove the cloves, bay leaves, and cinnamon sticks before serving.

Watercress Couscous

2 tablespoons olive oil
½ cup finely diced red onions
2 cloves garlic, minced
2 cups low-sodium vegetable or chicken broth
½ cup golden raisins
2 scallions, sliced
1 teaspoon sea salt, divided
1⅓ cups couscous
8 ounces cherry tomatoes, quartered (1½ cups)
2½ packed cups watercress, woody stems removed
2 tablespoons fresh lemon juice
½ teaspoon freshly ground black pepper

Watercress is one of the most nutritious leafy greens out there. This often-overlooked summer vegetable is chock-full of powerful nutrients, including vitamin K. A cup of watercress has a whopping 100 percent of the Recommended Daily Intake (RDI) for vitamin K, not to mention heart-healthy antioxidants. The first time I saw watercress at our farmers market, I fell in love with its delicate peppery taste. When it's in season I sprinkle it on everything I can for nutrition, color, and taste. This is such a delicious and beautiful, yet nutritious, dish. The subtle sweetness from the raisins and the slight peppery taste of the watercress come together so well with the added touch of fresh lemon juice. Of course if you can't find watercress you can easily substitute kale, arugula, or dandelion greens. This side dish is such a winner. Pair it with any of the mains, such as Shrimp and Tomato Stew with Scallions (page 190) or Tofu and Mushrooms Stir-Fry (page 235).

In a medium saucepan with a tight-fitting lid, heat the oil over medium heat. Add the onions and cook, stirring occasionally, until translucent, 4 to 5 minutes. Add the garlic and cook, stirring, for 30 seconds.

Add the broth, raisins, scallions, and ¾ teaspoon of the salt and bring to a boil over high heat. Stir in the couscous, cover, and remove from the heat. Let sit for 5 minutes without removing the lid.

Meanwhile, in a large bowl, toss together the tomatoes, watercress, lemon juice, remaining ¼ teaspoon of salt, and the pepper. Add the couscous and stir gently until combined. Serve.

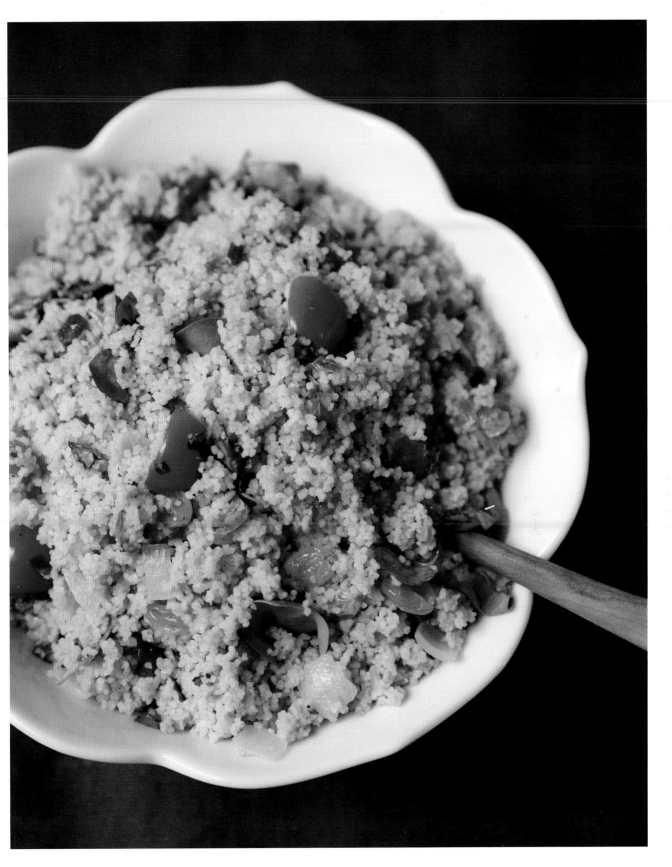

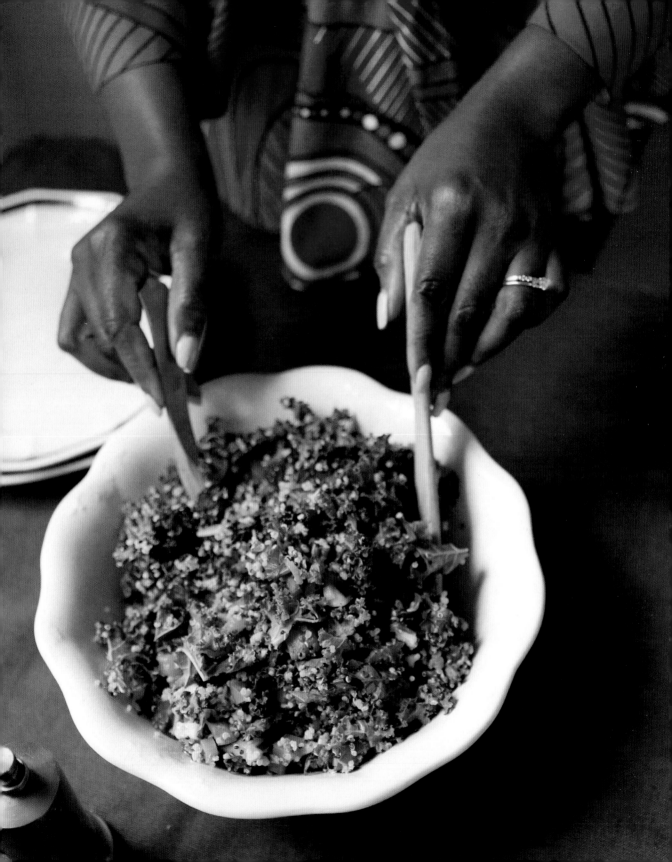

Everyday Kale Salad

½ bunch kale, stemmed and finely chopped (about 2 packed cups)

3 tablespoons fresh lime juice

2 cups low-sodium vegetable or chicken broth

1 small onion, finely diced

2 cloves garlic, minced

¼ teaspoon ground cumin

¼ teaspoon smoked paprika

1 cup quinoa, rinsed

½ cup diced tomatoes

½ cup diced yellow bell pepper

½ cup diced cucumber

4 scallions, thinly sliced

¼ cup minced fresh flat-leaf parsley

⅓ cup minced fresh basil

⅓ cup dried cranberries

⅓ cup toasted pecans, chopped

Sea salt

Freshly ground black pepper

Another name for this could be the "necessity is the mother of invention" salad, since that is how this dish happened. One day I was running on fumes, with little money or time to spare. All we had were a few bags of cooked quinoa, half a bunch of kale, half a cucumber, and a few cherry tomatoes. I put them all together and jazzed the mixture up with spices to feed my family that evening. I share this meal with you from a place of love and gratitude. There truly is no darkness without light. For the days that all seems lost, pull the little you have together. You will be surprised how deeply your family will enjoy it. While this dish was made from remnants, it is loaded with nutrients and healing herbs, is high in protein and fiber, and tastes absolutely delicious.

In a large bowl, toss together the kale and lime juice until evenly coated and set aside.

In a medium saucepan with a tight-fitting lid, bring the broth, onion, garlic, cumin, and paprika to a boil over medium heat. Add the quinoa, stir, and return to a boil, then reduce the heat and simmer, covered, for 7 minutes. Remove from the heat and let rest, covered, for about 20 minutes. Fluff with a fork and transfer to the bowl with the kale.

Add the tomatoes, bell pepper, cucumber, scallions, parsley, basil, cranberries, pecans, and season with salt and pepper to taste mix well, and adjust the seasonings as needed. Serve right away, or refrigerate, covered, up to a day.

3 tablespoons olive oil, divided
1 onion, thinly sliced
⅓ cup thinly sliced leeks, pale green and white parts
1 large carrot, peeled and julienned
5 cups thinly sliced green cabbage (about ½ head)
3 tablespoons apple cider vinegar
1 tablespoon maple syrup
2 tablespoons chopped fresh flat-leaf parsley
½ teaspoon sea salt
¼ teaspoon freshly ground black pepper

Warm Crunchy Coleslaw with Leeks and Carrots

This delicious mayo-free slaw is a go-to side in my house all year long. Cabbage is full of gut-friendly fiber, which helps keep the digestive system healthy and running smoothly. So if you are backed up, try eating more cabbage. If you aren't a fan of cabbage, give this recipe a try. You might be pleasantly surprised by how delicious such a simple dish can be. And here's a little kitchen hack for my picky eaters: I stuff this slaw into wanton wrappers and air fry them to golden crispy perfection, and I have yet to find a picky eater who turned it down. This side can be paired with any and every dish. The key is to slice your onions and leeks as thinly as you can so you do not bite down on big chewy pieces.

In a large skillet, heat 1 tablespoon of the oil over medium-high heat. Add the onion and leeks and cook, stirring occasionally, until the onion is translucent, about 5 minutes. Transfer to a large mixing bowl, reserving the skillet.

Add another tablespoon of oil to the skillet and reduce the heat to medium. Add the carrot and cook, stirring occasionally, until tender, about 3 minutes. Transfer to the onion bowl, reserving the skillet.

Add the remaining tablespoon of oil to the skillet over medium heat. Add the cabbage and cook, stirring constantly, until lightly wilted, about 3 minutes. Transfer to the onion bowl, reserving the skillet.

Add the vinegar and maple syrup to the skillet over medium heat, stir to combine until the mixture starts to bubble, about 30 seconds. Pour the mixture over the slaw, add the parsley, salt, and pepper and mix gently until thoroughly combined. Transfer the slaw into a large bowl and serve warm.

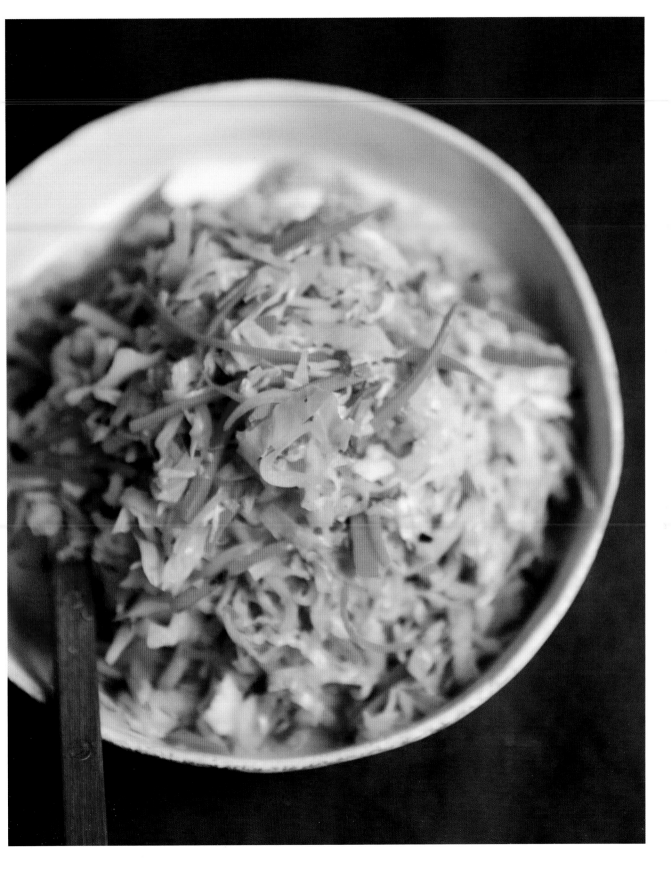

Chickpea and Cucumber Salad

This is the perfect refreshing, cooling side dish for a hot summer day. Along with chickpeas, which are high in protein, and cucumbers, it features tomatoes, jicama, and avocado in a super-lemony dressing. A little hack helps to keep this on rotation in my kitchen during the summer with very little effort: I cook a big batch of chickpeas in my pressure cooker and freeze them in 2-cup portions, making this dish so easy to pull together. This salad can honestly pair with any mains, including my favorites, Herb- and Parmesan-Crusted Chicken (page 173) and Tofu and Mushrooms Stir-Fry (page 235).

In a large bowl, combine the cucumbers, tomatoes, onion, chickpeas, avocado, jicama, and parsley.

In a small bowl, whisk together the olive oil, lemon juice, honey, mustard, garlic, salt, and pepper. Pour the dressing over the salad and stir very gently until evenly coated. Serve.

NOTE: Do not serve honey to babies twelve months or younger, as it may cause infant botulism. Use maple syrup instead.

2 cucumbers, finely diced
2 tomatoes, finely diced
1 small red onion, diced
2 cups cooked chickpeas, drained; if using canned, drained and rinsed
1 firm but ripe avocado, halved, peeled, pitted, and diced
1 cup finely diced jicama
⅓ cup chopped fresh flat-leaf parsley
¼ cup olive oil
Juice of 2 lemons
1 tablespoon raw honey (see Note)
½ teaspoon Dijon mustard
2 cloves garlic, minced
1 teaspoon sea salt
¼ teaspoon freshly ground pepper

SERVES 4 TO 6

Sautéed Green Beans and Carrots

I love the nutritional profile of this simple, delicious side. Green beans are chock-full of antioxidants that fight free radicals and help reduce cell damage. Green beans are also full of fiber. But the taste is what gets me every time. The combination of green beans and carrots with onions and tomatoes cooked in olive oil and their own juices is delicious. Serve alongside Beef Tenderloin with Rosemary and Thyme Potatoes (page 135) or Lemony Salmon Kebabs (page 198).

3 tablespoons olive oil
1 onion, diced
2 cloves garlic, minced
2 tomatoes, diced
2 scallions, thinly sliced
½ cup low-sodium vegetable or chicken broth
3 carrots (about ½ pound), quartered lengthwise and cut on the bias to match the length of the halved green beans
1 (1-inch) piece of fresh ginger, peeled and grated
½ teaspoon crushed red pepper flakes (optional)
½ teaspoon sea salt
½ pound green beans, halved on the bias
2 tablespoons minced fresh flat-leaf parsley

In a large skillet, heat the oil over medium heat. Add the onion and cook, stirring often, until translucent, about 5 minutes. Add the garlic and cook, stirring constantly, until fragrant, about 1 minute.

Add the tomatoes and scallions and cook, stirring occasionally, until the tomatoes begin to soften, about 7 minutes. Add the broth, carrots, ginger, red pepper flakes, if using, and salt and cook for 3 minutes. Stir in the green beans and parsley and cook, stirring occasionally, until tender, about 3 minutes more. Transfer to a medium bowl and serve.

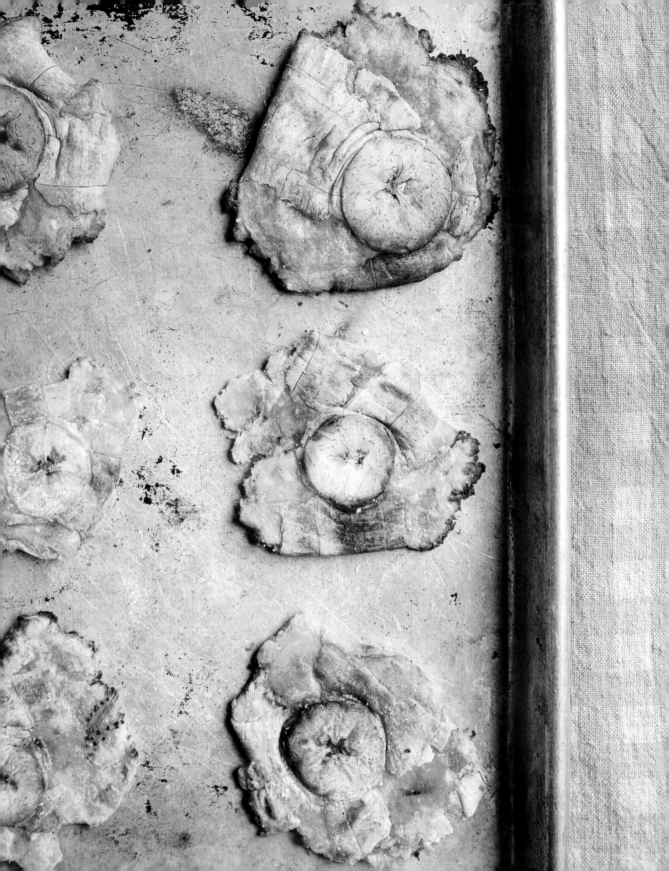

GF, DF

SERVES 2 TO 4

2 green (or semi-
  ripe, if you want a
  slight sweetness)
  plantains, peeled
1 tablespoon olive oil
½ teaspoon salt

Plantain Tapé

TWICE-FRIED PLANTAINS

Plantain Tapé is plantains that are fried in oil twice. You fry them for a few minutes, remove them from the oil, flatten them, and then fry them again to golden crunchy perfection. You will find a version of this childhood favorite in most African and Central and South American countries. The plantains are absolutely delicious fried, but they are just as good prepared in an air fryer and are certainly healthier. Plantains are an unsung hero in the U.S. They are chock-full of nutrients, fiber, and resistant starch, a prebiotic that promotes gut health. For those on a gluten-free diet, there is truly nothing you can't make with plantains. Plantain flour is gaining traction in North America as a wonderful single-ingredient replacement for wheat flour in baked goods, including pancakes and cakes. (Iya Foods is my go-to brand.)

Heat an air fryer to 375°F.

Cut the plantains into 3- to 4-inch slices depending on size. Place in the air fryer and cook until starting to brown, 5 to 7 minutes. Transfer to a cutting board, leaving the air fryer on, and flatten by placing slices upright and then pressing down on one at a time with the bottom of a plate. Drizzle with the oil and sprinkle the salt on both sides.

Return the flattened plantains to the air fryer in a single layer (depending on the size of the fryer, it might take a couple of batches) and cook until golden brown and crispy on the edges, flipping half way through, about 10 minutes. Serve.

NOTE: You can make the popular West African dodo (fried plantains) in an air fryer as well. To air fry green or sweet (ripe) plantains, quarter lengthwise, then cut into 1-inch cubes, season with a pinch of salt, drizzle with a little olive oil, and simply air fry.

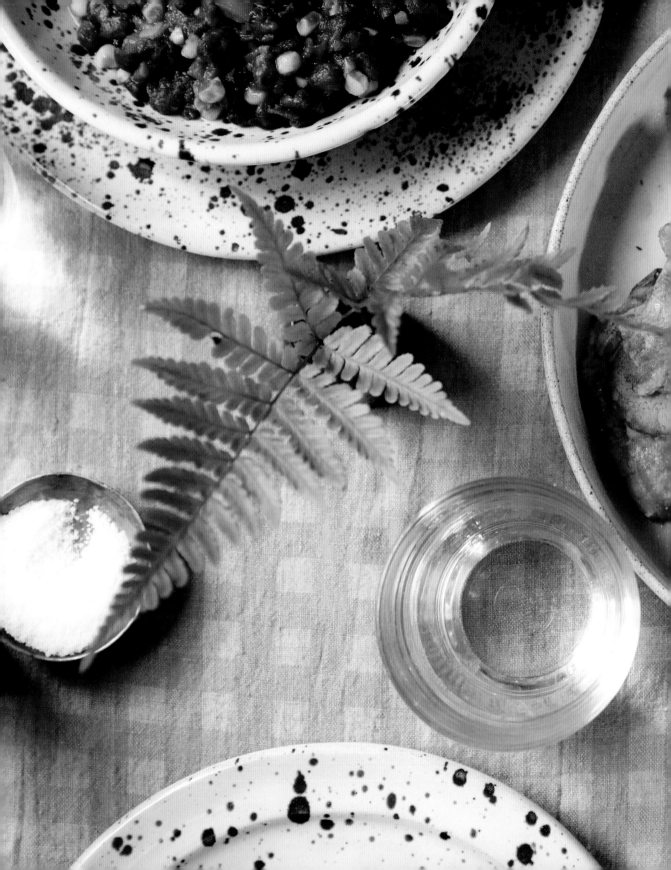

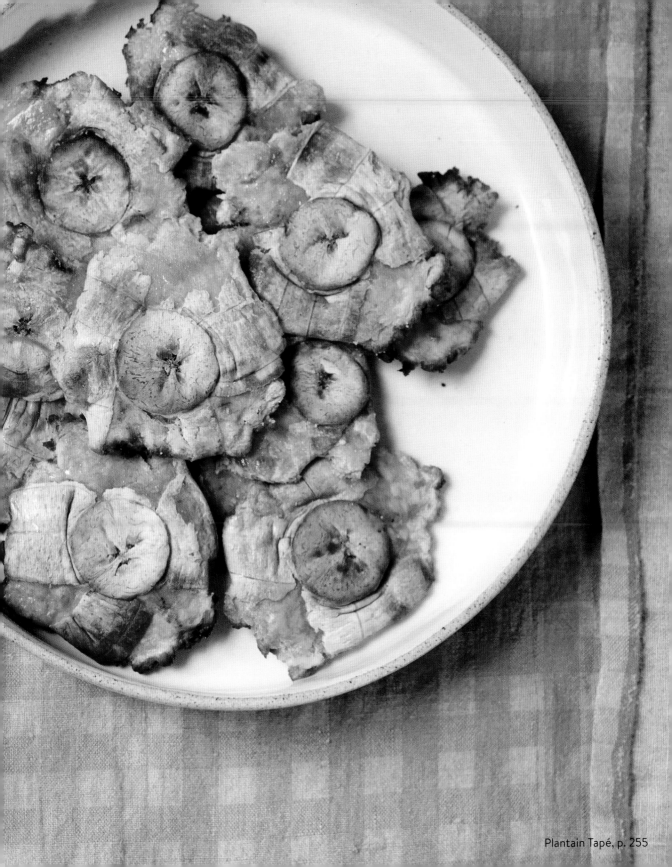

Plantain Tapé, p. 255

Herbed Parmesan French Fries

2 large russet potatoes, peeled and cut into ¼-inch-square sticks and soaked in ice water for 15 minutes
1 tablespoon olive oil
1 teaspoon minced fresh rosemary leaves
1 teaspoon minced fresh thyme leaves
1 teaspoon sea salt
⅓ to ½ cup freshly grated Parmesan cheese, preferably Parmigiano Reggiano
¼ cup finely chopped fresh flat-leaf parsleyv

The first time I made this recipe in the air fryer I posted it on Instagram. Actress and influencer Tamera Mowry-Housley shared it on her Instagram account and, within an hour, it had 44,000 likes. Looking at the pic, you would never guess there was no deep-frying involved. An air fryer produced those beauties! So, if you or your kiddos love fries, particularly fast-food fries, try this recipe instead. It's easy and so good! If your air fryer is small, make the fries in batches, then reheat all the fries together at 390°F (not a traditional temperature, but it works) until hot, 2 to 3 minutes.

Preheat an air fryer to 375°F.

Drain the potatoes and pat dry. In a large bowl, toss together the potatoes, oil, rosemary, thyme, and salt until thoroughly combined. Place the potatoes in the air fryer and cook for 10 minutes. Shake and flip the potatoes and cook until crisp, 6 to 8 minutes more.

Transfer the fries to a large bowl and sprinkle with the cheese and parsley, and a pinch of salt, if needed. Serve.

½ cup mayonnaise
1 clove garlic, minced
2 tablespoons ketchup
2 tablespoons finely
diced onion
1 teaspoon ground
turmeric
⅛ teaspoon freshly
ground black pepper
¼ teaspoon sea salt,
or to taste
1 teaspoon fresh
lemon juice

Turmeric Garlicky Mayo

This mayo not only jazzes up anything you put it on but also is chock-full of nutrients, with the addition of garlic and turmeric. Use homemade mayo or good-quality store-bought and never compromise taste. Pair this with any sides or mains. I love it with Black Bean Burgers (page 210). I have been known to simply eat it by itself on those days when life gets in the way and all I crave is comfort food.

In a small bowl, stir together all the ingredients, then refrigerate for up to 5 days.

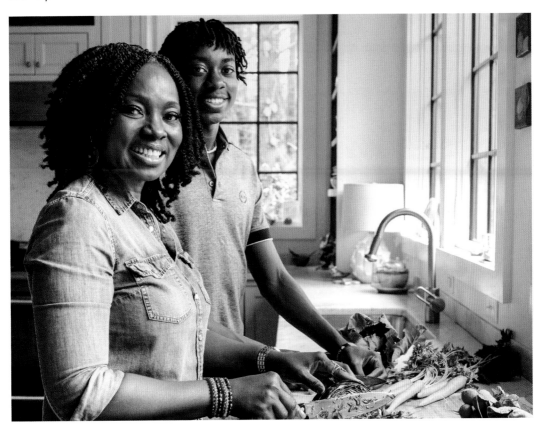

2 cups dried whole
    red chiles or ¾ cup
    crushed red pepper
    flakes
4 cloves garlic, divided
3 whole cloves
1 teaspoon sea salt
1½ cups avocado oil
1 cinnamon stick
3 star anise pods
1 onion, quartered
1 bay leaf
3 (½ × 2½–inch) slices
    fresh ginger
1 finely chopped
    scallion

All-Purpose Hot Sauce

My Chinese-inspired chili-oil sauce is the perfect compromise when it comes to hot sauce in my kitchen, and today it is a favorite with my guests and social media community. When I first moved to the United States, I learned really fast that not everyone likes or is even used to hot, fiery dishes, I needed to cook without adding Scotch bonnet pepper but wanted something that those of us who love it spicy could easily add to our food. While there are lots of hot sauces on the market, I find their taste a little vinegary, which changes the flavor profile of my dishes. This aromatic sauce, though not as hot as Cameroonian Scotch bonnet pepper sauce, is so tasty and doesn't have the tart taste of the American-style hot sauce. I also add fresh garlic and scallions, which take the taste a notch higher. I can't tell you how many jars of this we go through in a month in my home. I hope it brings you as much joy as it does me. Add it to any dish when you need to increase the heat deliciously.

Add the dried red chiles to a food processor and grind on high speed until they become small flakes.

Transfer the chile flakes into a large heat-proof bowl. (Be careful not to inhale here!) Mince 2 of the garlic cloves and add them to the same bowl, along with cloves and salt.

In a small pot, heat the oil over medium-low heat until hot. (Place a wooden chopstick inside the oil to check for bubbles to tell if the oil is hot.) Add the cinnamon, star anise, onion, bay leaf, remaining 2 garlic cloves, ginger, and scallion.

Allow to gently simmer for 30 minutes while stirring occasionally. Using a slotted spoon, remove and discard the aromatics.

Very carefully pour the hot oil into the heat-proof bowl and let it bubble. As it bubbles, stir the sauce to prevent the top from overcooking or burning.

Allow the mixture to cool. Transfer into an airtight glass jar and store in the refrigerator for up to 2 months.

Mashed Potatoes with Beets

GF

SERVES 4 TO 6

1½ pounds Yukon gold potatoes, peeled and quartered

1 small red beet, peeled and cut into ½-inch cubes

½ cup Cashew Milk (page 273) or Almond Milk (page 269)

6 tablespoons (¾ stick) butter

Sea salt

Freshly ground black pepper

I created these creamy mashed potatoes with beets for a super-picky eater who was also allergic to many foods. I hoped he would find the pink color irresistible, and it worked! I use nut milk here, but you can absolutely use regular milk if you prefer. Aside from the color and mild flavor, the beets—a nutritional powerhouse—add fiber, antioxidants, and natural nitrates, which can help lower blood pressure. Our youngest, who is seventeen years old, loves this side; he prefers this now over regular mashed potatoes because it looks beautiful and tastes amazing. Serve this in place of regular mashed potatoes any time.

Rinse the potatoes and beets and place them in a medium heavy-bottomed pot with just enough water to come halfway up their sides. Cover and bring to a boil over high heat, then reduce the heat and simmer until fork-tender, 20 to 25 minutes.

Drain the remaining liquid from the pot into a small bowl and set aside. Transfer the potatoes and beets to a medium bowl, reserving the pot. Add the milk and butter to the pot and gently heat until hot.

Pass the potatoes and beets through a ricer or drum sieve into the pot (or you can mash them by hand, but they won't be as smooth) and cream together with a spoon. Stir in the reserved liquid a few tablespoons at a time until you reach the desired consistency. Season with salt and pepper and serve.

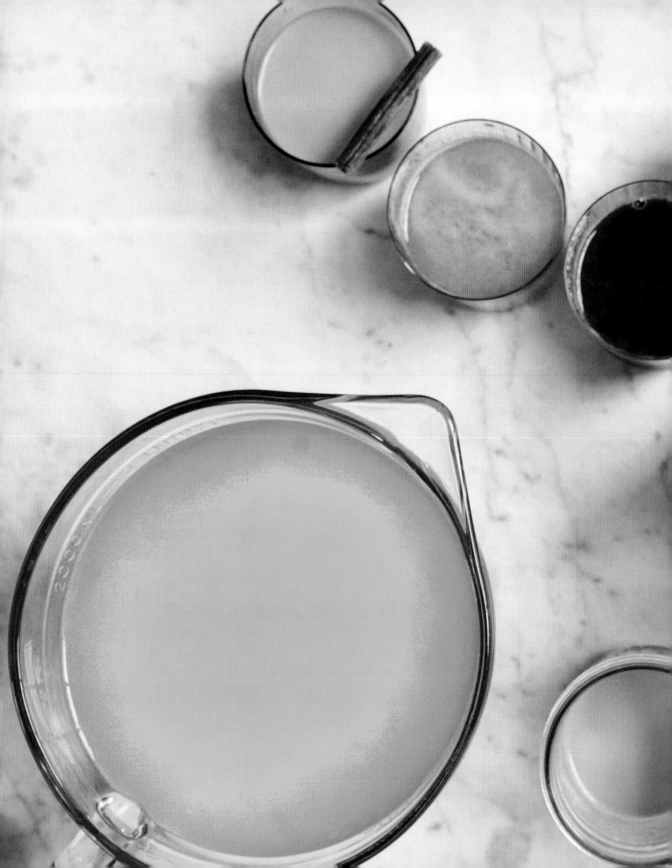

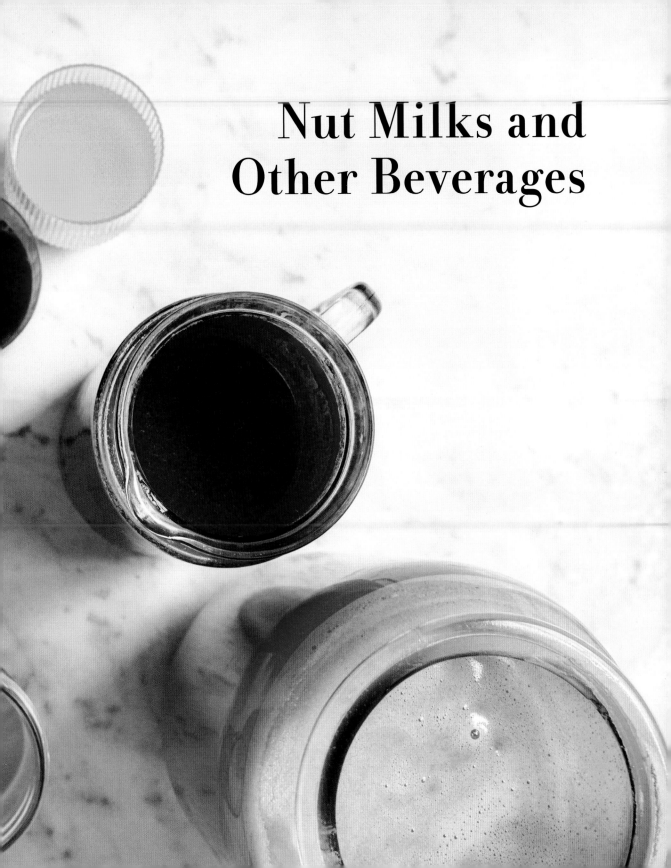

Nut Milks and Other Beverages

RICH IN ANTIOXIDANTS AND MONO- and polyunsaturated fats, dairy-free alternatives like nut and grain milks are a delicious and nutritious alternative to cow's milk. Commercial dairy-free milk alternatives are undeniably convenient, but the proportion of nuts or grains to other ingredients is fairly low.

For the most part, homemade milks are far superior in both quality and taste. They are also cheaper than store-bought. (There are a few brands of nut and grain milk that don't contain fillers or emulsifiers, but they are quite pricey.)

Some of my recipes in this book call for dairy-free milk. But when it comes to everyday consumption (in cereal, coffee, etc.), you don't have to be vegan to make the switch to nondairy milk. I advise my clients to limit their intake of dairy, especially for children, for many reasons. As a parent and health-care worker looking at scientific data all the time, I am frustrated by the USDA's call for three servings of dairy a day; that's a lot of dairy for human consumption. Aside from the realities of industrial dairy farming, dairy greatly decreases the body's absorption of iron, and it doesn't equal strong bones either. In fact, studies have shown that 165 milligrams of calcium from milk, cheese, or a supplement reduced iron absorption by 50 to 60 percent. That is problematic, as increased calcium intake is commonly recommended for children and women, the same populations that are at risk for iron deficiency.

Growing up in Bamenda, a province in the northwestern part of Cameroon, I drank raw milk. Do I go into a panic when my kids occasionally use dairy? The answer is a resounding no; we live for summer ice cream treats. When we are visiting family and friends and dairy is what they have, my only push is that it be organic and I call it a day.

Of course there are drinks beyond milk. As a mother and an integrative practitioner, I've always felt strongly about having a home that is free of soda and other sugary drinks. I know way too many adults who have tried to stop drinking them with very little success—even when their health depends on it. It has taken some serious effort and commitment on my part, along with putting up with tantrums when the kiddos were younger, to make this work. Now that my kids have gotten older, they really don't have a taste for those drinks. That said, it was always important to me to make sure my kids didn't feel deprived, so I created my own fun, tasty, and healthy drinks with simple, seasonal ingredients—nothing fake, nothing artificial. I hope you like them as much as we do.

My hope is that this information plants a little awareness bug in your ear to pay more attention and hopefully help you figure out how to make it all work for you and your family. This might mean you switch things up a little with some of the alternatives here. Dairy might become an occasional treat, as it is in our home. You might befriend a small local farmer pasture-raising and grass-feeding animals for some raw dairy. You might swap sodas for some of these drinks. However you chose to use this information I pray it is nothing but empowering to you and your family for generations to come.

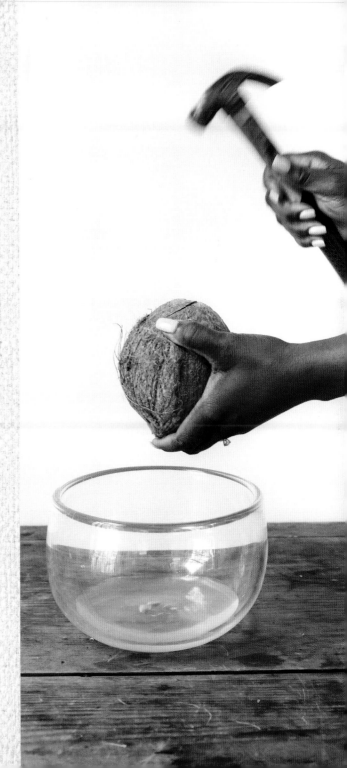

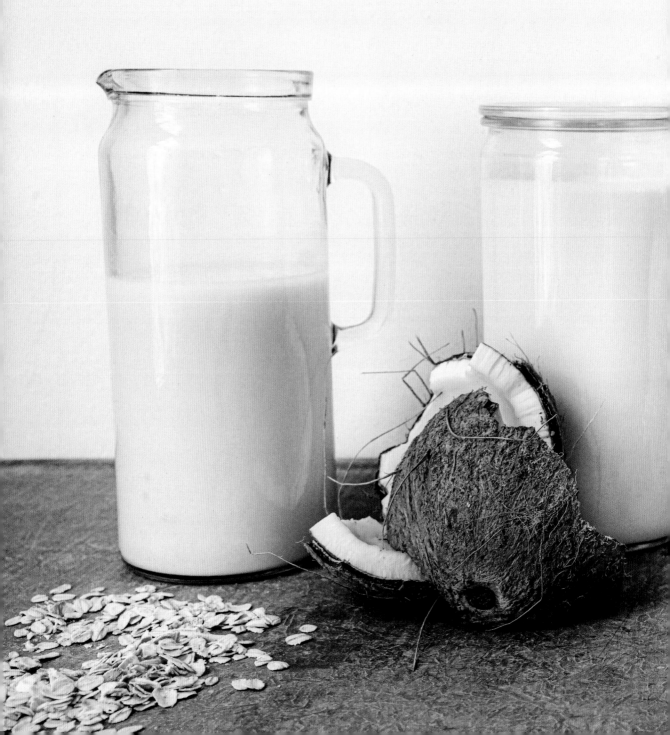

Oat Milk,
p. 274

Coconut Milk,
p. 270

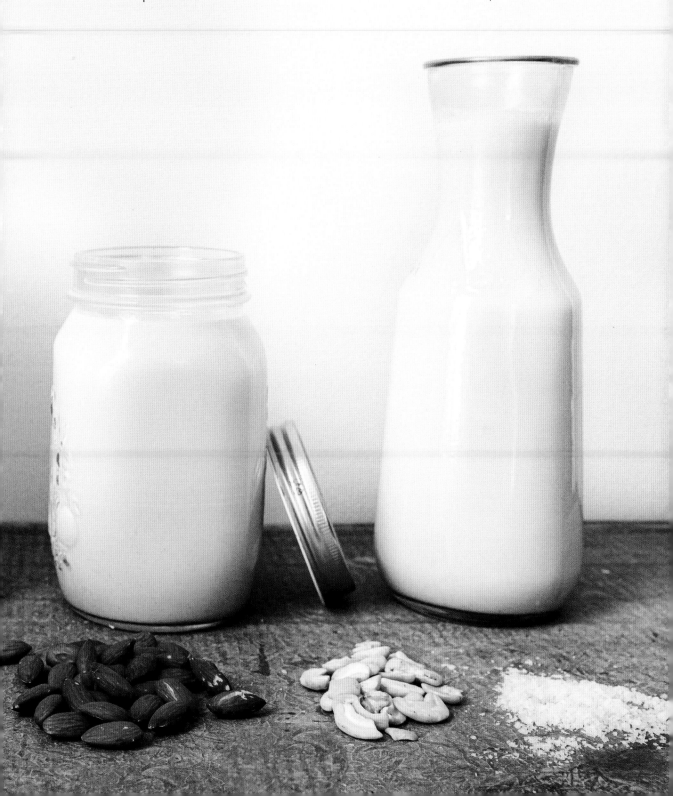

Almond Milk,
p. 269

Cashew Milk,
p. 273

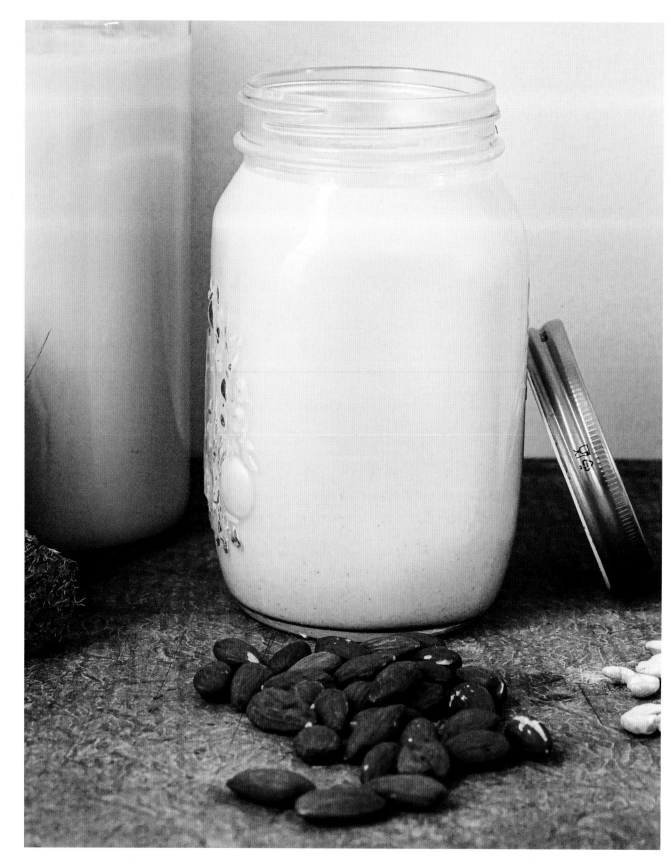

1 cup raw almonds,
    soaked in water
    overnight in the
    refrigerator
¼ teaspoon sea salt
3 to 4 cups water

Almond Milk

The first time you make your almond milk at home will be the day you
step back and ask yourself, "Why did it take me so long?" Homemade
almond milk tastes so much better than store-bought, boasts more
nutrients, and can be adapted to your needs at hand. I now make
creamer (using less water) for Georges's coffee, which he loves.
When you make your almond milk at home you also get to reuse and
repurpose any leftover pulp as you wish: you can make your own
almond meal, you can make crackers, or you can add the pulp to your
smoothie for more fiber.

Drain and rinse the almonds until the water runs clear. In a blender,
blend all the ingredients plus 3 to 4 cups water (for a thicker consistency,
use less water; for a thinner consistency, use more) until creamy, 1 to
2 minutes depending on your blender.

Strain the mixture through a strainer lined with cheesecloth and
set over a medium bowl or large jar. Carefully gather the corners of
the cheesecloth, lift it up, and gently squeeze until all of the liquid is
extracted.

Transfer the almond milk to an airtight container and refrigerate,
covered, for up to 4 days. (You can freeze the almond milk for up to
3 months, too!)

NOTES: A good high-powered blender makes a huge difference in getting as
much milk from your almonds as possible.

To flavor the milk, you can add 1 teaspoon vanilla extract, blend with
2 Medjool dates and/or 2 tablespoons maple syrup.

1 large brown coconut
2 to 3 cups warm water

Coconut Milk

I grew up making coconut milk for Coconut Jollof Rice (page 189): we would grate the coconut manually using a contraption similar to a box grater using the side with the smallest holes to get the most milk out of the coconut. Unlike almond milk, which I discovered in the U.S., I was already a connoisseur of coconut milk, and the store-bought kind wasn't it; it left my coconut jollof wanting. I saved up for a blender and haven't looked backed since. When you make your coconut milk at home, the quality and taste is so much better and it is way cheaper. An added bonus is the pulp: Don't throw it away; dry it and use any way you like.

Using a sharp knife or a screwdriver, pierce the 3 eyes of the coconut and drain the water into a bowl. (You can drink it or reserve it for another use.) Place the coconut on a hard surface lined with a kitchen towel (preferably a concrete surface; tile might crack!) and smack it with a hammer, meat mallet, or sturdy rolling pin until it splits open.

Using a paring knife, carefully pry the coconut meat from the husk. Rinse the meat and blend in a high-powered blender with the warm water until creamy.

Strain the mixture through a strainer lined with cheesecloth and set over a medium bowl or large jar. Carefully gather the corners of the cheesecloth, lift it up, and gently squeeze until all of the liquid is extracted.

Transfer the coconut milk to an airtight container and refrigerate, covered, for up to 4 days. It will separate over time, so stir before using.

NOTE: For a thicker consistency, use less water; for a thinner consistency, use more.

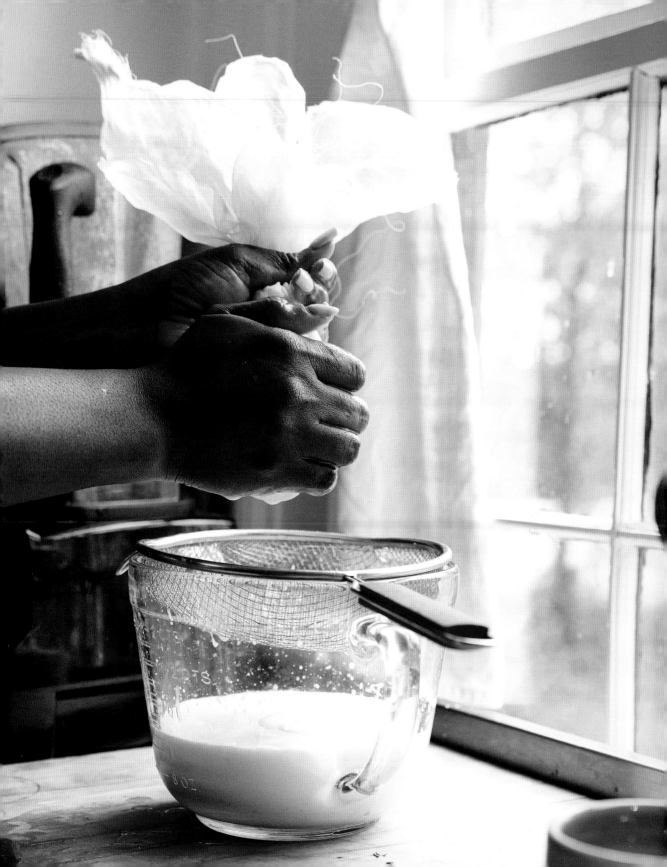

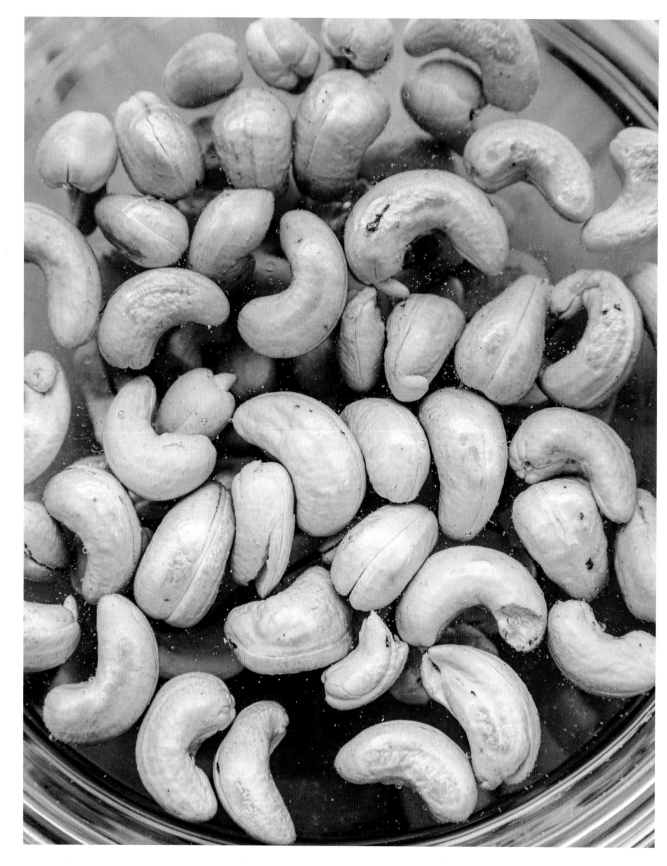

1 cup raw cashews,
soaked in water
overnight in the
refrigerator
3 to 4 cups water
1 to 2 tablespoons
maple syrup
2 teaspoons vanilla
extract
¼ teaspoon sea salt

Cashew Milk

Cashew milk is the silkiest milk of all nondairy milks to me, and when you experience it made from scratch, you will never want anything less than the best again, more so than with any other milk. It is chock-full of heart-healthy fats, protein, and a host of impressive vitamins and minerals. It is also the easiest milk to make if you have a high-powered blender, since it'll get silky without the need for cheesecloth.

Drain and rinse the cashews until the water runs clear. In a high-powered blender, blend 3 cups of water and the rest of the ingredients until soft, 1 to 2 minutes or longer, depending on the blender. Add the last cup of water and continue blending until the cashews are completely pulverized. If you want it thicker, start with 2 cups of water instead of 3.

Strain the mixture through a strainer lined with cheesecloth if you are not using a high-powered blender and set over a medium bowl or large jar. Carefully gather the corners of the cheesecloth, lift it up, and gently squeeze until all of the liquid is passed through (there usually is very little pulp left).

Transfer the cashew milk to an airtight container and refrigerate, covered, for up to 4 days. It will separate over time, so stir before using.

4 cups ice water
1 cup old-fashioned
   oats (see Note)
1 tablespoon maple
   syrup
1 teaspoon vanilla
   extract
¼ teaspoon sea salt

Oat Milk

Allergies and food intolerance are a huge problem in our society today, as many people can't consume either dairy or nuts. Oat milk is naturally free of many common allergens including lactose, making it a wonderful option. If you are one of the many who have been buying commercial oat milk, here is an opportunity for you to give homemade oat milk a chance. Of all the many nut and plant milks I have made, oat milk has been the trickiest: You have to be super careful not to overblend or you end up with a slimy concoction. I recommend investing in a good blender; with a high-powered blender you can actually use steel-cut oats to make your milk, too.

In a blender, blend the all the ingredients for 30 seconds; do not overblend.

Strain the mixture through a strainer lined with cheesecloth and set over a medium bowl or large jar. Carefully gather the corners of the cheesecloth, lift it up, and gently squeeze as much as you can without overdoing it—the more you squeeze the more chances of slime. (Save the pulp for baked goods or smoothies.)

Transfer the oat milk to an airtight container and refrigerate, covered, for up to 4 days. It will separate over time, so stir before using.

NOTE: For allergies and gluten intolerance make sure you are buying oats that are certified gluten-free.

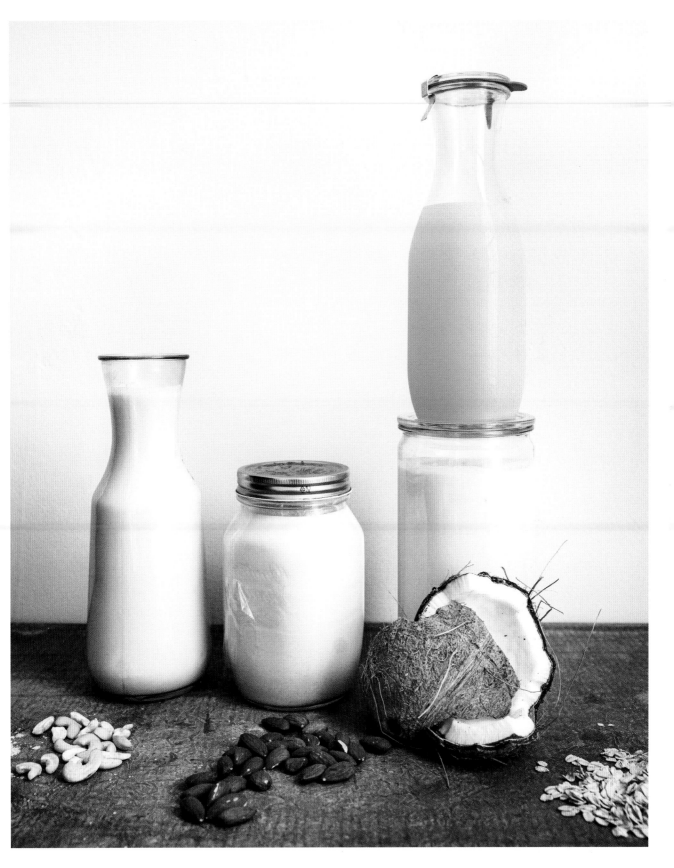

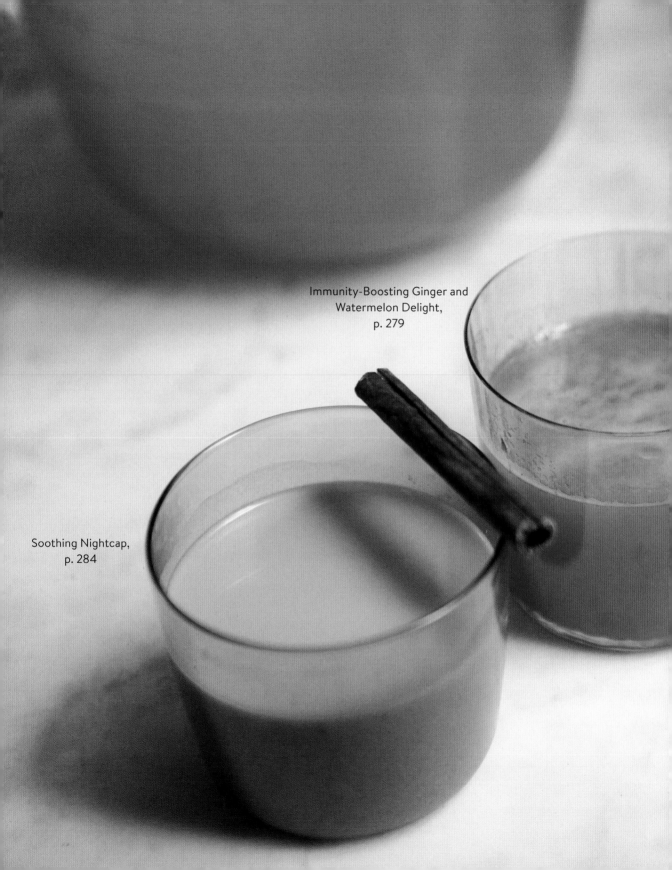

Immunity-Boosting Ginger and
Watermelon Delight,
p. 279

Soothing Nightcap,
p. 284

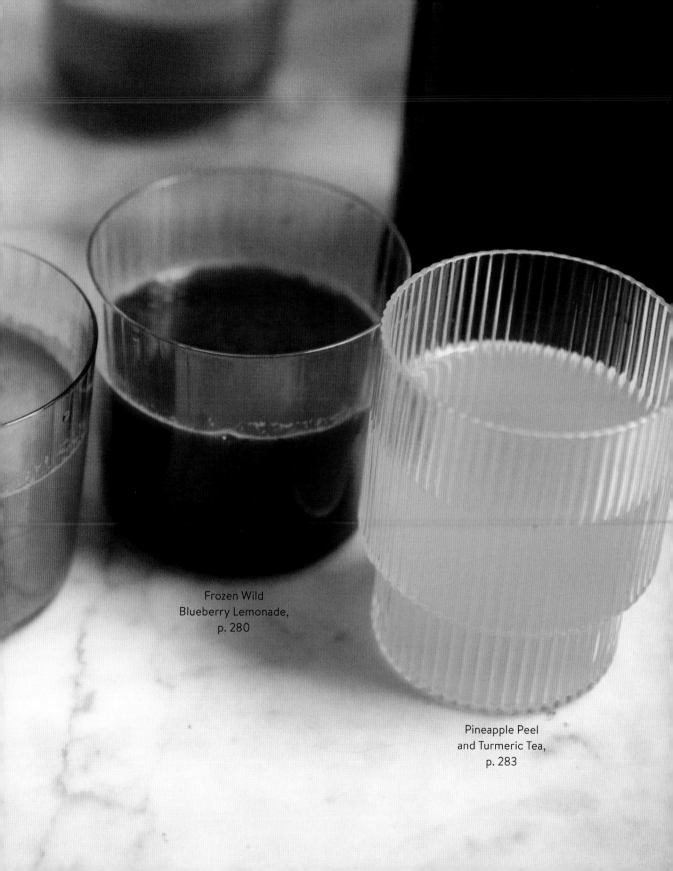

Frozen Wild
Blueberry Lemonade,
p. 280

Pineapple Peel
and Turmeric Tea,
p. 283

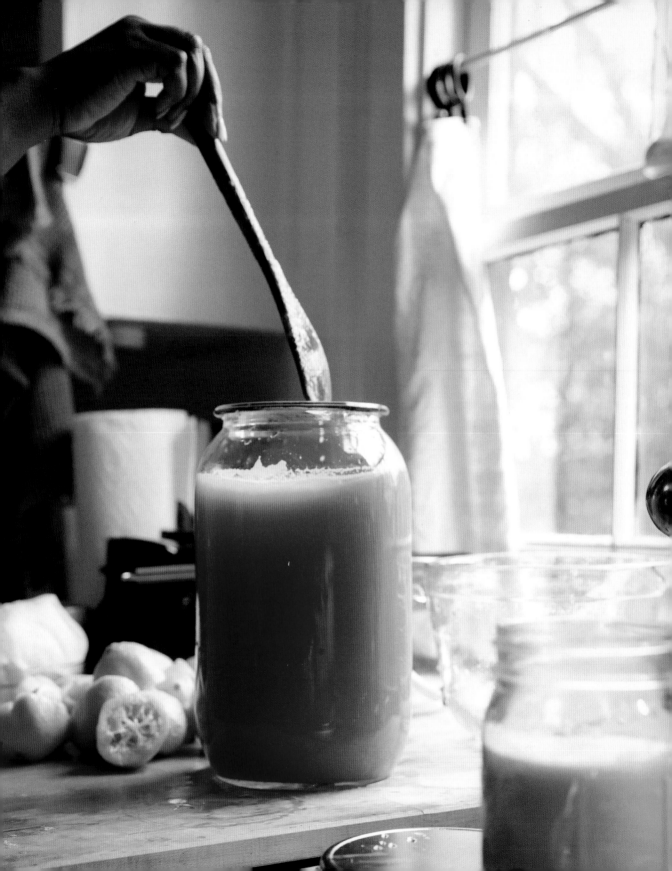

1½ pounds ginger,
  peeled
1 medium watermelon
  (will make 5 cups of
  juice)
2½ quarts water
Juice of 12 lemons
Raw honey, to taste
  (see Note)

Immunity-Boosting Ginger and Watermelon Delight

Georgia is as hot as it can get outside of my home countries of Nigeria and Cameroon, where it feels like the sun is resting on your roof. This is a nutritious drink that you will feel good about serving your family all summer long. Ginger is one of the world's oldest and most popular medicinal spices; its anti-inflammatory and antioxidant properties help boost immune-system health. With the antibacterial and antiviral properties of fresh lemon juice and the high potassium from the watermelon, this drink is a healthy option for the whole family, especially the kiddos. Of course kids just want their drink to taste delicious and look as vibrant as that of the kid next door, so this drink is a win for all. This recipe can be easily modified for smaller or bigger crowds; invest in reusable glass bottles to store in the refrigerator for up to 5 days, if it lasts that long.

In a food processor or blender, process the ginger until smooth. Strain the mixture through a strainer lined with cheesecloth and set over a medium bowl or large jar. Carefully gather the corners of the cheesecloth, lift it up, and gently squeeze until all of the liquid is extracted.

Cut the melon in half and use a big spoon to scoop out chunks. Place the fruit in a blender and blend until pulverized, strain using cheesecloth, if you are not a fan of pulp.

Stir in the water, watermelon juice, lemon juice, and honey to taste. Pour into jars with lids and refrigerate for up to 5 days. Shake, pour, and enjoy. It also makes an amazing base for adult drinks—try it with a splash of vodka.

NOTE: Do not serve honey to babies twelve months or younger, as it may cause infant botulism. Use maple syrup instead.

1½ cups frozen blueberries, preferably wild
½ cup raw honey (see Note)
8 cups water, divided
¼ cup fresh lemon juice

Frozen Wild Blueberry Lemonade

This is one of my all-time favorite summer drinks and I am so glad the kiddos love it even more. The beautiful, vibrant color and the refreshing taste from the combination of lemon, raw honey, and wild blueberries on a hot summer day is pure bliss. Wild blueberries are rich in antioxidants and anti-inflammatory properties. You can use regular blueberries, but, if you can, use frozen wild blueberries for their superior nutrients, vibrant color, and affordability. (They are cheaper than organic!) I sometimes use sparkling water to make it fizzy, which the kiddos love. Serve and watch their happy faces.

In a small saucepan, combine the blueberries, honey, and 1 cup of water. Bring to a boil over high heat, then lower the heat and gently simmer for about 5 minutes. Remove from the heat and let cool.

Strain the mixture through a strainer into a large container. (Save the blueberries for smoothies or pancakes.) Stir in the remaining 7 cups of water and the lemon juice and refrigerate until cold, about 2 hours, or for up to 5 days. Serve chilled.

NOTE: Do not serve raw honey to babies twelve months or younger, as it may cause infant botulism. Use maple syrup instead.

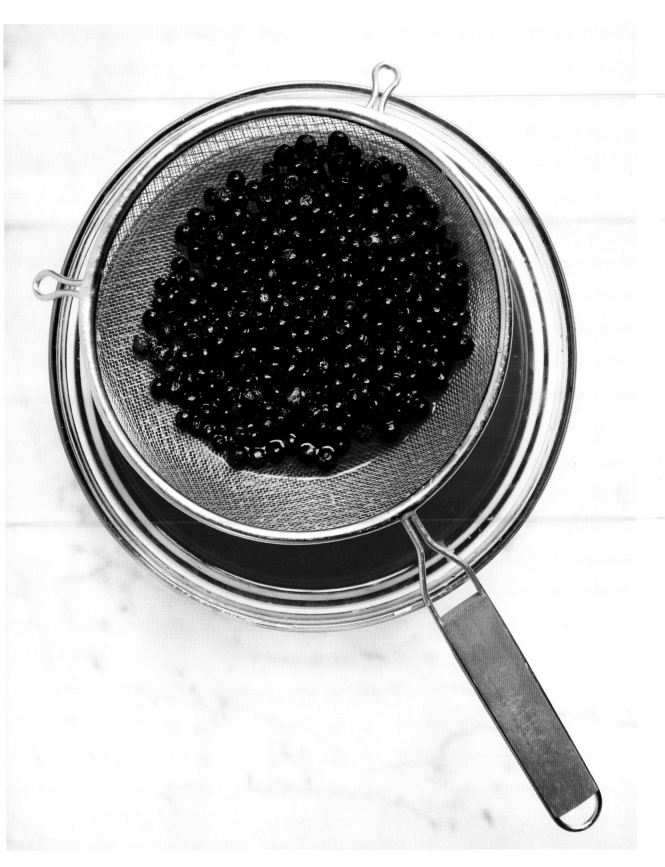

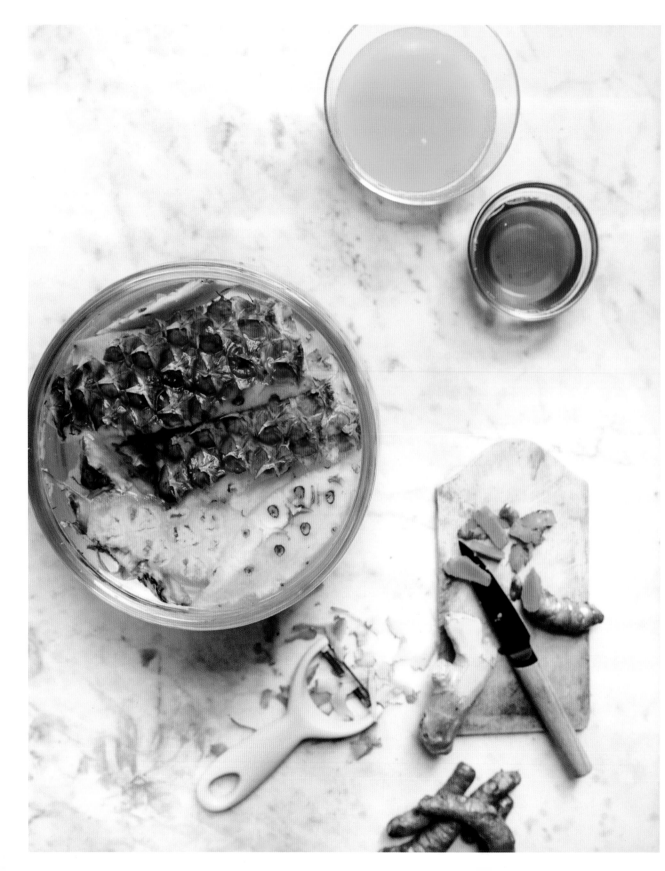

GF, DF

MAKES 16 CUPS

Peel and core of
  1 large pineapple
1 tablespoon apple
  cider vinegar
1 gallon plus 1 cup
  water
1 (2½-inch) piece
  fresh ginger, peeled,
  thickly sliced, and
  smashed
1 (2½-inch) piece
  fresh turmeric root,
  peeled, thickly
  sliced, and smashed
⅛ teaspoon freshly
  ground black pepper
Juice of 2 lemons
Juice of 2 oranges
3 tablespoons
  raw honey, or to
  taste (see Note)

Pineapple Peel and Turmeric Tea

Once you make this tea, you'll kick yourself for all the times you threw away the peelings after cutting up a pineapple. While the fruit itself is enjoyed around the world, not many people are aware of the health benefits of the trimmings. They are high in bromelain, a powerful enzyme known for its anti-inflammatory effects, as well as manganese and vitamin C, which are good for teeth and bones. They also aid indigestion and help with constipation. To make the tea, the peelings and core are boiled with ginger and turmeric and then the strained liquid is flavored with citrus juice, honey, and black pepper and chilled. It's a delightful, refreshing drink that can be enjoyed any time of the year but is best when pineapples are in season.

In a large pot, combine the pineapple rind (not the core) and enough water to cover. Stir in the vinegar and let soak for 30 minutes.

Meanwhile, bring the water to a boil over high heat.

Rinse the pineapple rind with fresh water, then carefully add the rind to the boiling water. Add the pineapple core, ginger, turmeric, and pepper, then return to a boil, reduce the heat, and simmer, covered, for 30 minutes. Let cool, then use tongs to remove and discard (or compost) the solids.

Whisk in the lemon and orange juice and honey to taste.

Strain the mixture through a strainer lined with cheesecloth and set over a medium bowl or large jar. Carefully gather the corners of the cheesecloth, lift it up, and gently squeeze until all of the liquid is passed through. (There usually is very little pulp left.) Refrigerate until cold, about 3 hours, or for up to 5 days. Serve chilled.

NOTE: Do not serve raw honey to babies twelve months or younger, as it may cause infant botulism. Use maple syrup instead.

Soothing Nightcap

1½ to 2 cups Coconut Milk (page 270)
2 tablespoons loose chamomile tea or 2 tea bags
¼ teaspoon grated peeled fresh ginger
¼ teaspoon ground turmeric
2 green cardamom pods
1 cinnamon stick
2 tablespoons raw honey (see Note)

If you are looking for a comforting, stress-relieving, delicious, and immunity-boosting drink outside of traditional hot cocoa, look no further. This creamy dairy-free drink, made with the healing benefit of turmeric, calming chamomile tea, tummy-soothing ginger, anti-anxiety properties of cardamom, and sweetened with raw honey, speaks nothing but healthy delicious comfort. I created this drink for our youngest when he was a kid; it is still a comfort drink to this day. While I love coconut milk and use it here, you are welcome to use any of your favorite dairy-free options.

In a small saucepan, bring the coconut milk, tea, ginger, turmeric, cardamom, and cinnamon to a simmer, whisking until combined. Keep just below a simmer, whisking occasionally, for 2 to 3 minutes. Remove from heat and allow the tea to steep for 2 minutes more.

Strain through a fine-mesh strainer into a small saucepan and whisk in the honey until the mixture is nice and frothy. Pour into 2 or 3 mugs and serve hot.

NOTE: Do not serve raw honey to babies twelve months or younger, as it may cause infant botulism. Use maple syrup instead.

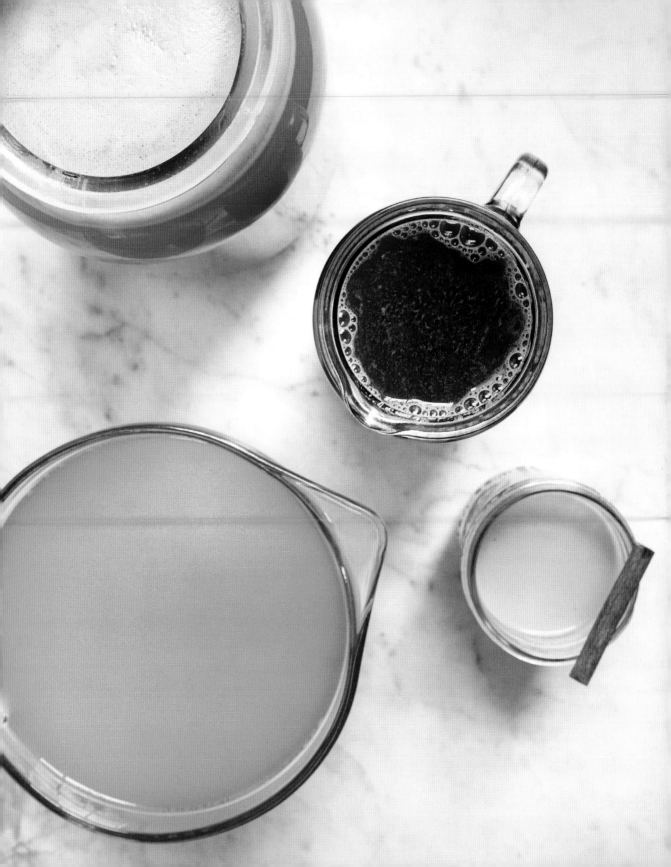

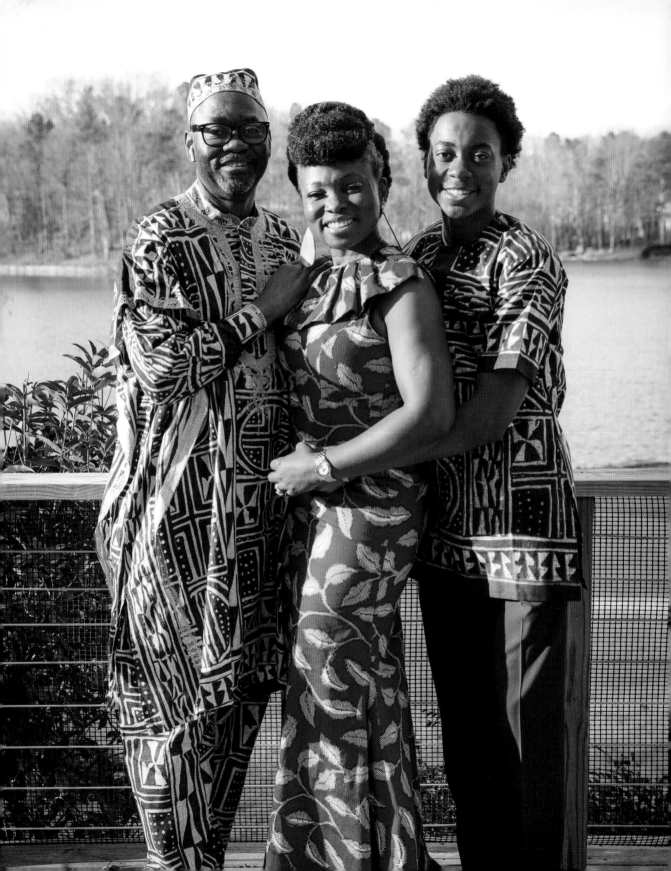

ACKNOWLEDGMENTS

I WISH TO THANK EVERYONE WHO contributed to this project. I am forever grateful for your help in bringing *Bountiful Cooking* to life.

So many amazing, creative people worked with me on this book. Rinne Allen, thank you for the gorgeous food photographs, you brought my vision to life so vibrantly, for pouring your gift into this project, from styling each and every plate to fit the mood and scene in my mind all the while filling your studio with laughter.

Big thanks to the most fun prep cooks Pete Amadhanirundr, Ally Smith, and *the* Hugh Acheson. I am still tickled that Hugh Acheson, cookbook author, chef, and restaurateur extraordinaire, was humble enough to be a part of my prep team. You guys made cooking away from home fun.

Andrew Lee, you are a genius, thank you for pointing your lens on me, you blew the cover shoot out of the water. And thanks to Alison Latimore and Yonah Wienges for capturing some behind-the-scenes footage.

Thanks to my unfailingly supportive agent and forever cheerleader, Alison Fargis, and to my incredible editor, Renee Sedliar, I'm grateful for your friendly guidance and crystal clarity. And to the rest of the team at Hachette—Alison Dalafave, Amanda Kain, Terri Sirma, Melanie Gold, and copyeditor Dorothea Halliday—you made writing this book such a beautiful and joyful experience, and my heart thanks you all.

Special thanks to Sara Bliss, for connecting the dots, forever grateful.

To my PR team, very special thanks go to Emerald-Jane Hunter, Sharon Kunz, and Ashley Kiedrowski.

My assistant, Grace Ehiosune, with magical fingers, you blessed me at a time when I needed it the most.

And thanks to all my family and friends who show up day in and day out, sometimes on very short notice, to help with photo shoots, read and reread manuscripts, conduct polls, and everything in between. For all the times you moved your schedules around to accommodate me, my Oga Georges Achindu, my #1 cheerleader and supporter, for always being there the past twenty years in marriage, and my brother Michael Chibili, there is no way I would have written this book without you both. Evelyn Ntiege, Sherri Sims, Dr. Yvonne Edjua, Dr. Euphrates Kinge, Victorine Fonjungo, Cheryl Wilson, Denene Millner, Ekene Onu, April and Carson Lake (and family), Audrey Forka, Viola Brumskine, Bianca Rhyme, Karolina Morsilo, Ify Okoh, Luvvie Ajayi Jones, and Sarah Palin Chaplin.

Thanks to my friend Ghazaleh Coulter for contributing her childhood recipe; Tami Ramsay, for letting me play in her kitchen while in Athens; Sydney and Derek, the beautiful couple at Ladybird Farm, for allowing us to harvest the freshest produce from their garden; Kevin Scollo at Independent Bakery, for the most wholesome, delicious breads; and Noah Brendel at Seabear for coming through with the mandoline.

Thank you to the thousands of mamas I have been fortunate to work with over the years, those who made it to my workshops or private sessions, to my thousands of friends on social media crying for a cookbook with every recipe shared, and most of all my son Jared-Zane, taster extraordinaire, and all the other tasters who have sat at and continue to grace my table.

And to everyone who has supported and inspired me along the way, though I can't list you all, I thank you and carry you in my heart with me.

INDEX

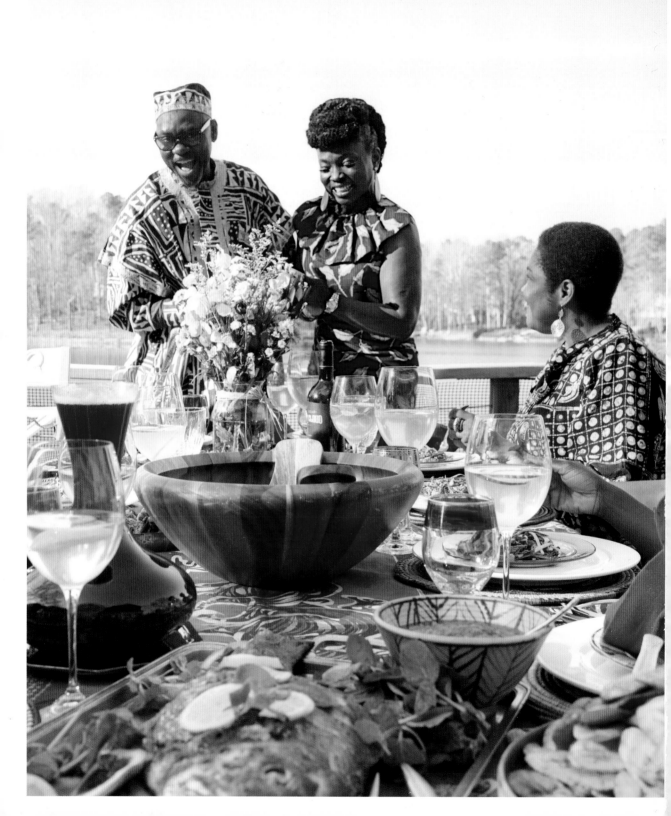